Common
Gynaecological
Conditions

Common Gynaecological Conditions

Patricia C. Wilson

**Blackwell
Science**

© 1999 by
Blackwell Science Ltd
Editorial Offices:
Osney Mead, Oxford OX2 0EL
25 John Street, London WC1N 2BL
23 Ainslie Place, Edinburgh EH3 6AJ
350 Main Street, Malden
    MA 02148 5018, USA
54 University Street, Carlton
    Victoria 3053, Australia
10, rue Casimir Delavigne
    75006 Paris, France

Other Editorial Offices:
Blackwell Wissenschafts-Verlag GmbH
Kurfürstendamm 57
10707 Berlin, Germany

Blackwell Science KK
MG Kodenmacho Building
7–10 Kodenmacho Nihombashi
Chuo-ku, Tokyo 104, Japan

First published 1999

Set by Excel Typesetters Co., Hong Kong
Printed and bound in Great Britain
at the University Press, Cambridge

The Blackwell Science logo is a
trade mark of Blackwell Science Ltd,
registered at the United Kingdom
Trade Marks Registry

DISTRIBUTORS

Marston Book Services Ltd
PO Box 269
Abingdon, Oxon OX14 4YN
(*Orders*: Tel: 01235 465500
        Fax: 01235 465555)

USA
Blackwell Science, Inc.
Commerce Place
350 Main Street
Malden, MA 02148 5018
(*Orders*: Tel: 800 759 6102
        781 388 8250
        Fax: 781 388 8255)

Canada
Login Brothers Book Company
324 Saulteaux Crescent
Winnipeg, Manitoba R3J 3T2
(*Orders*: Tel: 204 837-2987)

Australia
Blackwell Science Pty Ltd
54 University Street
Carlton, Victoria 3053
(*Orders*: Tel: 3 9347 0300
        Fax: 3 9347 5001)

A catalogue record for this title
is available from the British Library

ISBN 0-632-05174-4

Library of Congress
Cataloging-in-publication Data

Wilson, Patricia C.
    Common Gynaecological Conditions /
Patricia C. Wilson.
        p.   cm.
    ISBN 0-632-05174-4
    1. Gynecology—Handbooks, manuals,
etc.   I. Title.
    [DNLM: 1. Genital Diseases, Female
handbooks.   2. Women's Health
handbooks.   WP 39 W752c 1999]
RG110.W54   1999
618.1—DC21
DNLM/DLC
for Library of Congress   98-46285
                                              CIP

For further information on
Blackwell Science, visit our website:
www.blackwell-science.com

Contents

Preface

The purpose of this book is to provide the busy doctor or health care professional with an easy reference manual for the diagnosis and management of common gynaecological conditions. So much has changed and advanced in recent years, and keeping up to date is a real problem for many practitioners. Bacterial vaginosis, the Mirena® intrauterine system (IUS), transdermal matrix hormone replacement therapy (HRT) patches, intracytoplasmic sperm injection (ICSI) and transcervical resection of the endometrium (TCRE) are conditions, devices or procedures that were unheard of just a few years ago. The public obtains information on new developments in health care from the media and the Internet almost before we get the chance to open our journals and digest their contents.

Despite all these exciting and innovative advances, the main core of gynaecological practice is made up of simple conditions that can occur commonly and fill up our clinics week after week. Their correct diagnosis and management are very important in the restoration of the health and well-being of the average woman, yet, frequently, misdiagnoses occur, e.g. the diagnosis of 'thrush' or a urine infection when the patient has genital herpes, or the prescription of norethisterone for the control of menorrhagia when no trial has shown a clear benefit.

This book has been organised in a synoptic manner to highlight common conditions with suggestions for diagnosis and clinical management. The chapters on HRT and fertility are fuller because this is a burgeoning field in gynaecological care and the array of treatment options can be bewildering to those who are not specialists in the field. It has been a challenge to write, and would not have been possible without the good humour and support of all my patients whose conditions appear in the book and who allowed me to photograph them in out-patients and during surgery.

Patricia C. Wilson FRCOG

Acknowledgements

I should like to pay tribute to the theatre team at The Rivers Hospital, Hertfordshire, and especially to Dr Ralph Robinson, Consultant Anaesthetist, and Mr Alan Williams, Senior ODA. They demonstrated endless patience and good humour, and developed remarkable photographic expertise, even with the lights off, in the operating theatre.

The clinic nurses, especially June Stannard, were enthusiastic and helpful.

When out-patients were being photographed, Richard Masters developed the pictures with great skill, and Eleanor Tanner typed the manuscript and introduced good ideas.

My family have endured a gynaecological invasion of their home with text and photographs. They are relieved that the book has been 'born' so that meals can once more be taken without the table being covered in gynaecological script.

I should like to thank the following colleagues for script reading, correction and advise on content.

Dr Sally Hope MA BM BCh MRCGP, *General Practitioner, Woodstock*

Dr Susan Horsewood-Lee MB BS MRCGP, *General Practitioner, London*

Mr David Horwell FRCOG, *Consultant Obstetrician and Gynaecologist*

Professor Michael Hull MD FRCOG, *Professor of Reproductive Medicine and Surgery, University of Bristol*

Professor Roger Jones MA DM FRCP FRCGP, *Wolfson Professor of General Practice (UMDS)*

Dr Caroline Marfleet, *Consultant in Reproductive Health Care and Family Planning*
Dr Peter Nutley BA MB BS DRCOG, *Barrister-at-Law and General Practitioner.*

Last, but not least, my patients have been wonderful in their cooperation and delight in being asked to participate. And I thank them all.

Patricia C. Wilson FRCOG

List of abbreviations

CIN	Cervical intraepithelial neoplasia
COCP	Combined oral contraceptive pill
CT	Computed tomography
DVT	Deep vein thrombosis
EUA	Examination under anaesthesia
FBC	Full blood count
FSH	Follicle stimulating hormone
GUM	Genitourinary medicine
HCG	Human chorionic gonadotrophin
HPV	Human papilloma virus
HRT	Hormone replacement therapy
HSG	Hysterosalpingogram
HVS	High vaginal swab
IUD	Intrauterine contraceptive device
IUS	Intrauterine system
IVU	Intravenous
LH	Luteinising hormone
LLETZ	Large loop excision of the transformation zone
MRI	Magnetic resonance imaging
MSU	Midstream urine
NSAID	Nonsteroidal anti-inflammatory drugs
PCA	Patient controlled analgesia
PID	Pelvic inflammatory disease
POP	Progesterone only pill
PV	Per vaginum
STD	Sexually transmitted disease
TCRE	Transcervical resection of the endometrium
TFT	Thyroid function test
UTI	Urinary tract infection

1   Vaginal and vulval problems

Vaginal discharge in young women

Bacterial vaginosis

The commonest cause of a non-itchy discharge is *bacterial vaginosis*.

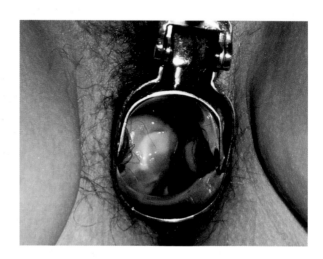

Fig 1.1 Profuse, non-itchy, offensive, grey discharge.

Incidence
10–30% of women can develop this at some stage in their lives. Sexual partners are not affected.

Aetiology
An overgrowth of anaerobic organisms at the expense of Lactobacillus, the acidic commensal of the vagina.

Symptoms
1 A discharge that stains underwear.
2 The discharge is not itchy.
3 An unpleasant malodorous, fishy smell — worse after sexual intercourse or menstruation.

Vaginal discharge in young women

Diagnosis

1 By history and speculum examination which reveals an adherent, thin, grey discharge.
2 The test of choice is a Gram stain of an air-dried sample of discharge. Glass slide sent to laboratory.
3 The usual high vaginal swab (HVS) has no place in the diagnosis.
4 Vaginal pH becomes alkaline (over 4.5). Special, narrow-range litmus paper is needed and can be ordered from: BDH Laboratory Supplies, Poole, Dorset, BH15 1TD.

Treatment

1 Metronidazole, either 2 g immediately or 400 mg twice daily for 7 days.
2 Clindamycin, 2% vaginal cream daily for seven applications.
3 Repeat courses of treatment may be required as 80% of women experience recurrences within 9 months.

Special points

1 Anaerobic bacteria produce amines which emit a fishy odour, and enquiry of this symptom may be a diagnostic pointer.
2 Intrauterine contraceptive device (IUCD) use may be associated with recurrent bacterial vaginosis.

Vaginal discharge in young women

Vulvovaginitis

The commonest gynaecological condition in the prepubertal child is *vulvovaginitis*.

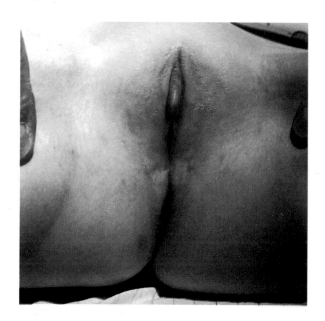

Fig 1.2 Inflammation and discharge found in recurrent vulvovaginitis.

Incidence
The most common cause of referral to the paediatric gynaecologist for girls between 3 and 7 years of age.

Aetiology
1 Oestrogen levels are low between birth and puberty, and the vaginal mucosa is thin, alkaline and has poor resistance to bacterial invasion.
2 Proximity of the anus with frequent perineal contamination of the vaginal orifice with bowel pathogens.
3 Poor perineal hygiene in children.

Vaginal discharge in young women

Symptoms

1 Inflammation and discharge with pain and pruritus.
2 Mother notices discharge on underwear.
3 Teacher may report child is rubbing herself or is uncomfortable in vulval area.
4 Nocturnal scratching and irritation suggest threadworm infection.
5 A bloodstained or offensive discharge suggests foreign body in vagina, but this is very rare.

Diagnosis

1 Inspection on mother's lap or on back with legs flopped open shows redness and discharge.
2 There may be *very little abnormality* to see on examination.
3 Introital swab usually grows non-specific organisms.
4 Midstream urine (MSU) to exclude urinary infection.
5 Examination under anaesthesia (EUA) is rarely indicated unless bleeding is also occurring.

Management

1 Strong reassurance to anxious parents.
2 Reassurance that it is self-limiting.
3 Prevention by thoroughly cleaning after bowels opened and wearing cotton underwear.
4 Avoid underclothes in bed and thick tights.
5 A bland skin cream, e.g. E45®, applied daily, can be protective.

Vaginal discharge in young women

6 Oral metronidazole can be given intermittently if discharge is offensive.

Special points

1 Candidiasis is rare in this age group and antifungals should *not* be prescribed or used by the mother on her child.
2 Distress to mother and child is intense and much reassurance is needed.
3 Fear of accusations of sexual abuse may deter the parent from seeking medical advice.

Candidiasis (thrush)

The commonest cause of an itchy discharge is *candidiasis* or *thrush*.

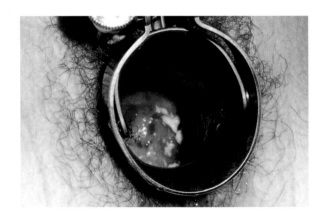

Fig 1.3 Curdy, adherent plaques and mucosal erythema.

Incidence
1 Accounts for 30% of vaginal infections.
2 Sexual partner may become infected and cause reinfection.

Vaginal discharge in young women

3 Many women self-medicate with antifungals available 'over the counter' so that the true incidence is unknown.

Aetiology
Caused by *Candida albicans*, but rarer forms such as *Candida glabrata* now appearing.

Symptoms
1 Thick, curdy, white discharge.
2 Intense vulval pruritus and itching.
3 Red, oedematous labia.
4 Perianal involvement.

Diagnosis
1 By speculum examination and history.
2 Confirm with an HVS sent to the laboratory in Stuart's medium.

Treatment
Initiate on history with any of the following.
1 Clotrimazole (Canesten®), as cream or pessary.
2 Fluconazole (Diflucan®), one 150-mg oral tablet.
3 Itraconazole (Sporanox®), 200 mg twice for 1 day.
If sexual partner has balanitis or postcoital symptoms, treat as well and advise use of condom. Cream-based antifungals are soothing to inflamed tissue and useful for the male partner.

Vaginal discharge in young women

1 Clotrimazole (Canesten®).
2 Miconazole (Gyno-Daktarin®).

Common misconceptions
1 The oral contraceptive pill is not implicated as an aetiological factor.
2 Threads of an intrauterine contraceptive device (IUD) do not predispose to infection.
3 Tight underwear does not cause thrush.
4 Natural yoghurt vaginal applications are of no proven benefit.

> **Special points**
>
> Often, women with primary herpes are initially diagnosed as having thrush and given antifungal treatment. If there is any doubt, refer to the genitourinary medicine (GUM) clinic for swabs and viral culture.

Recurrent candidiasis

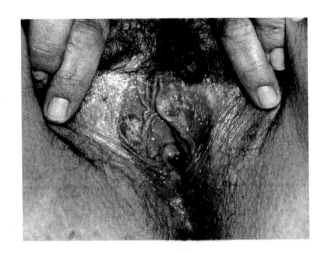

Fig 1.4 Spongy, erosive *Candida* with perianal spread.

Vaginal discharge in young women

Incidence
One per cent of women present with recurrent attacks which can be monthly.

Aetiology
1 Virulent strains of *Candida* (*glabrata*).
2 Predisposition to infection by changes in cell-mediated immunity.
3 Deep infiltration of the vaginal epithelium by *Candida* hyphae suggests that infection may not be superficial and this may be a factor in chronicity.

Symptoms
1 Repeated debilitating attacks of discharge and vulval pruritus often related to sexual intercourse and the menstrual cycle.
2 White, spongy areas on perineum and labia.
3 Red erosions from itching and chronic infection.
4 Perineal and perianal spread and itching.
5 Apareunia resulting from 'sexual intercourse-induced' attacks.

Diagnosis
1 Persist with swab taking as before to prove that *Candida* is at fault.
2 Patient can swab her vagina and send swab in before starting medication.

Treatment
Repeated drug therapy to suppress the attacks for *at least 6 months* with any of the following.

Vaginal discharge in young women

1 Clotrimazole (Canesten®), 500-mg single-dose pessary 1 week before and 1 week after menstruation for 6 months.
2 Fluconazole (Diflucan®), 150-mg oral tablet on first day of menstruation for 6 months.
3 Itraconazole (Sporanox®), 200 mg orally on first day of menstruation for 6 months.
There is no evidence that prolonged courses of 14 days of treatment are more effective than short courses.

Special points

1 So-called 'anti *Candida*' diets that eliminate sugar, yeasts and dairy products from the diet have not been proven to be effective in any clinically reported trial.
2 Diabetic women are particularly 'at risk' of chronic thrush vulvitis.

Physiological vaginal discharge

The commonest cause of an excessive, clear discharge is an *ectropion of the cervix* (often referred to as an *erosion*).

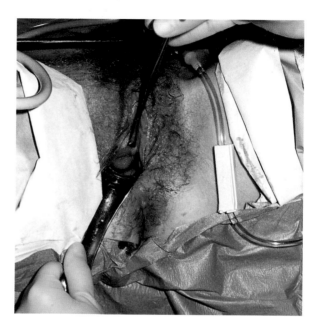

Fig 1.5 Large, red ectropion of the cervix.

Incidence
Five per cent of women will report an excessive, clear discharge at some stage in their lives to their GP.

Aetiology
1 The oral contraceptive pill and the pregnant state induce columnar epithelium to spread over the transformation zone. Columnar epithelium is secretory.
2 Mild chronic cervicitis with mixed bacteria can develop in the transformation zone.

Physiological vaginal discharge

3 Excessive mucous secretion and nabothian follicle formation. The cervix is composed of dense glandular epithelium which is more active in some women.

Diagnosis
1 With Cusco speculum, a large, red, mucous area on the cervix will be seen.
2 Thick, clear or white strands of mucus can be seen pouring out of the cervix.
3 The patient complains of feeling 'wet' and having to change underwear several times a day. Many wear a 'pantie pad' daily.

Treatment
1 Exclude cellular abnormality with a smear.
2 HVS to exclude infection and treat if necessary.
3 Cautery as an out-patient with a coagulator. Recurrence of symptoms may occur.

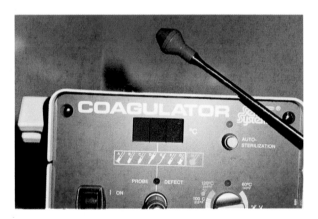

Fig 1.6 Coagulation as an out-patient is simple and painless.

Vaginal discharge in the older woman

The commonest causes are *atrophic vaginitis* and *poor vulval hygiene*.

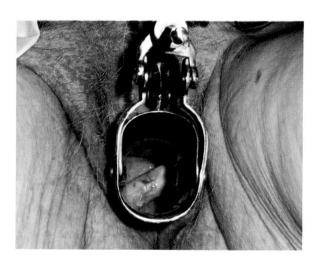

Fig 1.7 Neglected ring pessary *in situ.*

Incidence
Not common, but any offensive discharge should be regarded as pathological in older women. They are embarrassed by the symptoms and often use harsh detergents to clean the vulva.

Aetiology
1 Atrophic vaginitis with poor vulval hygiene.
2 Infection or ulceration with a ring pessary.
3 Genital malignancy.

Symptoms
Often concealed by fear and the hope that it will go away.

Vaginal discharge in the older woman

1 Staining of underwear.
2 Unpleasant vaginal odour.
3 Erratic bleeding with micturition or defaecation.

Diagnosis
1 Good visualisation of the vagina and cervix by speculum examination to exclude a tumour.
2 Swab and cervical smear if indicated.
3 Assessment of uterus by ultrasound may be necessary.
4 Simple atrophic vaginitis appears as thin tissue with multiple, small, red bleeding points when touched or scraped by the speculum blade.

Treatment
1 Genital tract malignancy must be excluded and gynaecological referral may be necessary to do this.
2 Ring pessary abrasions respond to ring removal and local oestrogen therapy and antibiotics, e.g. oestriol (Ortho-Gynest®) pessaries and amoxycillin and clavulanic acid (Augmentin®), one, orally, three times daily for 7 days.
3 Simple atrophic vaginitis can be treated with topical oestrogen, e.g. oestriol (Ortho-Gynest®) pessaries, one **PV** *nocte* for 2 weeks, and can be used intermittently to maintain vaginal health.

Special points

1 Vaginal examination in the elderly can be difficult because of stenosis and introital contracture.
2 An EUA may be necessary to exclude malignancy and to make a confident diagnosis.

Vulval pain in young women

Genital herpes

The commonest cause of vulval pain and ulceration in general practice is *genital herpes*.

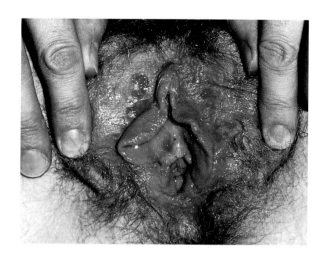

Fig 1.8 Genital ulceration caused by herpes virus.

Incidence
1 Increasing worldwide and accounts for about 5% of GUM clinic referrals.
2 About 4–5% of the population carry the virus usually from herpes simplex virus (HSV) I (cold sore) inoculation as a child.

Aetiology
1 HSV I and II.
2 Sexually transmitted, often with orogenital contact.
3 The primary attack usually results from sexual intercourse with a partner who is a carrier with *asymptomatic shedding*.
4 Primary attacks may occur in stable, long-

Vulval pain in young women

standing relationships where the seropositive partner has not had any symptoms.

Symptoms
1 Intensely painful vulva about 5 days after contact.
2 Dysuria and even retention of urine.
3 Small, red blisters and ulcers on labia.
4 General malaise and flu-like symptoms.
5 Groin lymphadenopathy.

Diagnosis
1 By history of intense pain.
2 By visual examination.
3 Confirm viral infection by swabbing the blisters or ulcers with a wet cotton tip swab and send to laboratory in a viral culture bottle. Request bottles from local laboratory.
4 Patients should be encouraged to attend their local GUM clinic to have the diagnosis confirmed and to screen for other sexually transmitted diseases (STDs).
5 Some may refuse and the GP can adequately manage the condition.

Treatment
Commence medication as soon as suspected with any of the following.
1 Aciclovir (Zovirax®), 200 mg five times daily for 5 days.
2 Famciclovir (Famvir®), 250 mg three times daily for 5 days.
3 Valaciclovir (Valtrex®), 500 mg twice daily for 5 days.

Vulval pain in young women

Counselling
1 Extremely important.
2 Patients feel angry, frightened and isolated by the diagnosis.
3 They need support and help from people with a positive attitude towards the infection.
4 Refer to GUM clinic if:
    (a) patient is willing (some are not);
    (b) patient is pregnant;
    (c) recurrent cases and non-responders.

Follow-up visit
Very important to discuss further management with regard to the following.
1 Viral transmission to future partners—viral shedding can occur randomly and without warning symptoms. Sexual partners should be made aware, but this is difficult and emotionally distressing for many women.
2 Contact lens wearers should exercise care as corneal infection can occur.
3 Pregnancy—attacks near to term may warrant a caesarean section for delivery.
4 Recurrent attacks are usual, and advice on how to recognise and manage them can be given.
5 Concomitant sexual infections can occur and screening should be advised.

Vulval pain in young women

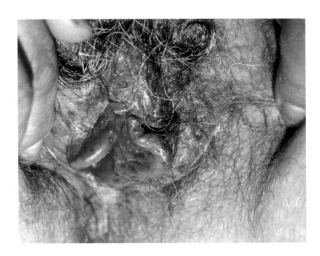

Fig 1.9 Healing, shallow ulcers of recurrent attacks.

Recurrent attacks

50–75% of patients will have recurrences.

1 May occur several times a year and often associated with stress, menstruation or trauma.

2 Less painful than the primary attack.

3 May be associated with extragenital lesions, e.g. skin, and patients will be infectious to partner.

4 If frequent and distressing, can be treated in the prodromal phase of tingling and discomfort with any of the following:

(a) aciclovir (Zovirax®), 400 mg twice daily for 5 days;

(b) famciclovir (Famvir®), 125 mg three times daily for 5 days;

(c) valaciclovir (Valtrex®), 500 mg twice daily for 5 days.

Vulval pain in young women

Suppressive therapy

1 Reserved for severely affected patients and those with psychosexual problems relating to recurrent attacks.

2 Medication as above should be given for 16 weeks and will be expensive.

Patient guide leaflet

What Do You Know About Genital Herpes? — Smith Kline Beecham.

Patient support group

The Herpes Virus Association, 41 North Road, London, N7 9DP. Telephone: 0171 609 9061.

Special points

1 Patients should abstain from sexual intercourse during attacks as the risk of transmission is high.

2 Half of patients will have asymptomatic viral shedding and can infect partners.

3 Women without antibodies to HSV I and II are particularly susceptible to infection from asymptomatic shedders.

4 Condom use may not protect against partner infection.

Vulval pain in young women

Vestibulitis

An important cause of intense introital pain in young, sexually active women.

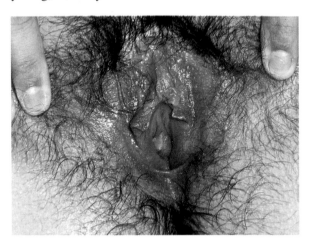

Fig 1.10 Red introitus and intense pain on pressure.

Incidence
Increasingly diagnosed now that it is recognised as a clinical entity in young women.

Aetiology
1 Unknown.
2 Was thought to be triggered by chronic infection with thrush, wart virus or bacterial vaginosis, but no consistent aetiological agent has been identified.
3 Inflammation of the minor vestibular glands occurs.

Symptoms
1 Fairly acute onset of intense introital or vaginal pain associated with pressure, tampon insertion or sexual intercourse.
2 Reddish, inflamed appearance, but non-specific changes around introitus.

Vulval pain in young women

3 Dyspareunia and even apareunia.
4 Strong emotional overlay with a psycho-sexual component.

Diagnosis
1 By history.
2 Gynaecological referral for confirmation, explanation and support recommended.

Treatment
1 The condition tends to resolve with time and no treatment modality shows a clear advantage at the present time.
2 The severe psychological overlay requires time and counselling. Patients feel that 'nobody can do anything to help'. Psychosexual problems develop and partners need to be involved.
3 A variety of treatments with lubricants, anaesthetic cream (Xylocaine 5% cream) and steroid cream (Dermovate®) are used to help the patient recover.
4 Very rarely, extreme cases may need surgical resection of the vestibule.

Special points
1 The condition is easy to diagnose because of the intense introital pain and dyspareunia, and hard to cure.
2 Much reassurance and support are needed.
3 Will eventually resolve.

Vulval pain in young women

Bartholin's cyst/abscess

A common cause of unilateral vulval pain and/or swelling.

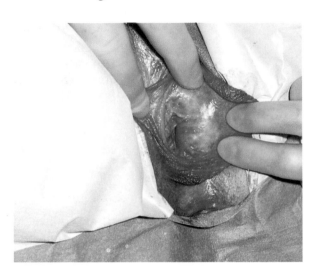

Fig 1.11 Enlarged cyst in posterolateral vaginal wall, left side.

Incidence
Frequent presentation to the GP in young women, often as an emergency if it becomes infected.

Aetiology
Paired Bartholin's glands open into the posterior introitus and secrete glairy mucoid lubrication prior to sexual intercourse. Blockage of the long, narrow duct leads to retention and often infection of the secretion.

Symptoms
1 A painless, cystic lump best felt by palpation. May increase and decrease in size.
2 Abscess formation with extreme pain if infection with introital organisms occurs.

Vulval pain in young women

Treatment
1 Referral for marsupialisation if uncomfortable.
2 Antibiotics and referral for drainage if infected.
3 Interval cystectomy may be required for recurrent infections.

Vulval pain in the older woman

Lichen sclerosis

The commonest cause of vulval discomfort in older women is *lichen sclerosis*.

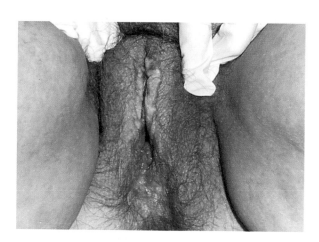

Fig 1.12 Lichen sclerosis — 'white skin'.

Incidence
Can occur in young women, but commonest in women over 60 years of age.

Aetiology
A dermatological change of unknown aetiology.

Vulval pain in the older woman

Symptoms
1 Intense vulval itching and pruritus.
2 Severe scratching, often in bed at night, and
even while asleep.
3 Cracked, abraded skin with bleeding.
4 Dyspareunia.
5 Strong emotional overlay develops.

Diagnosis
Easy diagnosis by visual inspection.
1 White, atrophic 'cigarette paper' skin.
2 Purpura and small blood blisters.
3 Tissue destruction with introital contracture,
resorption of labia minora, clitoral phimosis and
perianal spread.
4 Biopsy of edge of lesion in out-patient clinic
will confirm diagnosis, but not always necessary.

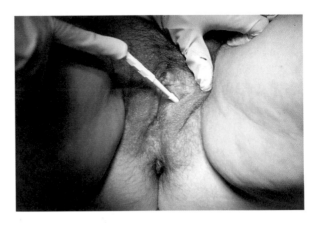

Fig 1.13 Biopsy.

Treatment
1 Use of a potent steroid ointment, clobetasol

Vulval pain in the older woman

propionate (Dermovate®), three times a day, and reducing after 1 month to twice a day and then once a month.

2 Caution about prolonged steroid use in this condition is inappropriate.

3 A 3-month treatment is required and maintenance with an emollient, such as Aqueous Cream, can be used. Repeated courses of self-medication to control symptoms is safe, but yearly review should take place.

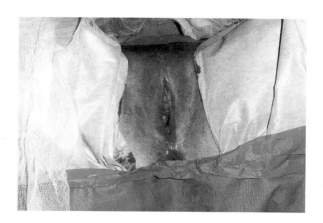

Fig 1.14 Note loss of labia minora and clitoral regression.

Long-term sequelae

1 Contraction of the introitus.
2 Loss of labial tissue.
3 Clitoral regression.
4 Apareunia.
5 Perineal cracking.
6 5% of patients may develop squamous cell carcinoma. Look for nodules or lumps at yearly review and refer for biopsy.

Vulval pain in the older woman

Special points

1 Patients are often prescribed oestrogen cream for this condition in the belief that it is an atrophic oestrogen condition. Oestrogen is ineffective and inappropriate.

2 The response to Dermovate® is rapid, and patients are very grateful for the amelioration of their misery, in particular night discomfort and scratching.

3 One of the most satisfying conditions to treat.

2   Menstrual disorders

Amenorrhoea — primary

The commonest cause of primary amenorrhoea (never had a period) is *primary ovarian failure* resulting from a chromosomal abnormality.

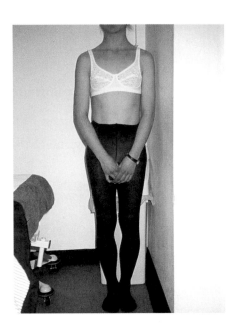

Fig 2.1 A 16-year-old school girl with primary amenorrhoea and weighing 40 kg.

Incidence
Not common, but occasional reason for consultation.

Aetiology
1 Chromosomal abnormality, e.g. Turner's syndrome, with streak ovaries 45, X0 or mosaic forms (45%).
2 Hypothalamic dysfunction from stress,

Amenorrhoea — primary

anorexia, hyperprolactinaemia and physical training (30%).
3 Anatomical abnormality — imperforate hymen (18%). Normal secondary sexual characteristics.

Management
1 Lack of breast development by the age of 14 years requires early investigation with follicle-stimulating hormone (FSH) and prolactin assay.
2 No periods by the age of 16 years requires referral to specialist gynaecological clinic for pelvic ultrasound and chromosomal studies.
3 Reassurance to anxious parents and the girl, and explanation if possible.

Treatment
1 Weighing and advice on diet and exercise to the small, thin girl.
2 Induction of secondary sexual development by hormone replacement therapy (HRT) may be considered in the specialist clinic.

Amenorrhoea — primary

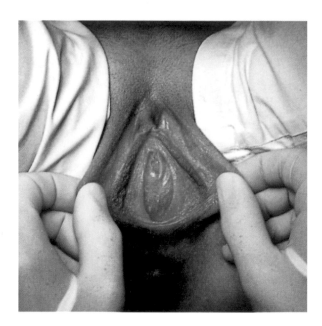

Fig 2.2 The 'imperforate hymen' is associated with normal secondary sexual characteristics. Reproduced from Leibowitch M, Staughton R, Neill S, Barton S, Marwood R. *An Atlas of Vulval Disease: A Combined Dermatological, Gynaecological and Venereological Approach*, 2nd edn, 1997, London: Martin Dunitz, with permission from the publishers.

3 Referral for surgical hymenectomy.
4 HRT for patients with Turner's syndrome to allow normal sexual development.

Special points

1 Most girls with Turner's syndrome are diagnosed at birth, and good gynaecological care involves supervision of HRT or the combined oral contraceptive pill (COCP) from the age of 13 years.
2 Underdeveloped and underweight girls are often reluctant to increase their weight as a thin physique is fashionable.

Amenorrhoea—secondary

The commonest cause of secondary amenorrhoea (cessation of periods for 6 months) is *excessive exercise or dieting* after pregnancy is excluded.

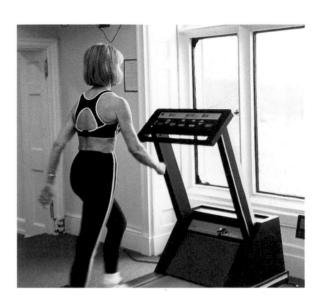

Fig 2.3 Intensively training sportswomen may develop amenorrhoea and osteoporosis with stress fractures.

Incidence
10% of young women may present with this symptom at some stage.

Aetiology
1 Pregnancy—often catches out the unwary!
2 Weight loss and/or excessive exercise, 38%.
3 Polycystic ovaries, 26%.
4 Premature or perimenopausal state, 22%.
5 Hyperprolactinaemia, 11%.

Diagnosis
1 Weight and height measurement.

Amenorrhoea — secondary

2 History to include diet, exercise, menstrual pattern, hot flushes, galactorrhoea and hirsutism.

3 Investigations:

(a) exclude pregnancy;

(b) serum FSH and luteinising hormone (LH) concentrations;

(c) serum prolactin and thyroid-stimulating hormone (TSH);

(d) pelvic ultrasonography to check for polycystic ovaries and endometrial thickness;

(e) refer if history longer than 6 months, or earlier if FSH or prolactin raised.

Management and treatment

Weight loss-induced amenorrhoea

1 The patient must understand that she has self-induced the condition.

2 Normal FSH and LH levels are present with oestrogen deficiency.

3 A threshold weight of about 47 kg is necessary for menarche and maintenance of menstrual flow.

4 Amenorrhoea can result when 10 kg of body weight is lost.

5 Dietary supervision is necessary, with increased calorie intake and regular weighing to encourage required weight to be achieved.

6 Barrier methods of contraception until periods resume or progestogen-only pill.

Amenorrhoea — secondary

Special points on anorexia nervosa

1 This is a serious, debilitating eating disorder that affects 1% of teenage girls, and may be a response to the psychosexual pressures of adolescence.

2 Half of all teenage girls feel that they are fat and need to diet. Peer group pressure is intense. Cosmetic dieting can lead to anorexia.

3 Rapid weight loss is often associated with psychological disturbance, and bulimia may develop. This is self-imposed starvation in a normally hungry person.

4 The mother may notice the girl developing food 'fads', spurning many sorts of foods for 'health reasons' and avoiding company at meals. Bingeing, vomiting and laxative abuse may be skilfully hidden. Depression, constipation and amenorrhoea develop. Treatment is based on psychiatric assessment and counselling with long-term supervision. Family support is essential.

5 It may persist into adult life with bizarre eating habits concealed, and carries a high morbidity and mortality rate.

6 Anorexic women are prone to osteoporosis in later life as dietary deficits in early years prevent maximum bone mass from being achieved by the third decade. HRT is needed if the underlying psychological disorder cannot be corrected to prevent early fractures.

Polycystic ovaries

The patient may have obesity, acne, hirsutism and infertility, as well as amenorrhoea.

Amenorrhoea — secondary

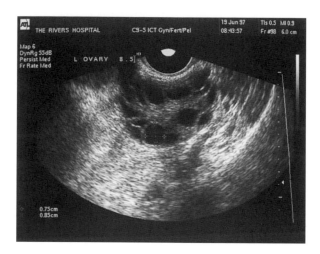

Fig 2.4 The 'necklace' effect of small follicles around the periphery of the ovary.

Special points

These women are well oestrogenised and can develop endometrial hyperplasia and even endometrial carcinoma in later life. Protection can be given by the use of the oral contraceptive pill, e.g. Dianette®.

1 Pelvic ultrasound scan confirms the 'necklace' effect of peripheral oocytes in 90% of cases.
2 Raised LH level over 10 IU/l in 60% of cases and raised 'free testosterone index'.
3 Overweight women should diet, but this can be impossible.
4 20% of women with this condition will ovulate and can conceive normally.
5 Dianette® is useful for contraception and control of hirsutism until fertility is required.
6 Fertility can be restored by using clomiphene citrate, 50 mg Day 2 to Day 6 of the cycle, to induce ovulation in 80% of women.
7 Non-ovulators will need specialist referral.

Premature menopause
Ovarian failure occurring before the age of 40 years, and associated with symptoms of hot flushes and vaginal dryness in previously normal women.

Amenorrhoea — secondary

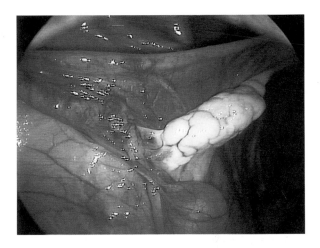

Fig 2.5 Crenated and shrunken appearance of the menopausal ovary.

1 The ovaries have usually 'run out of eggs'.
2 Diagnosed by a raised FSH over 30 IU/l on three occasions.
3 If pregnancy is desired, 'donated eggs' will be required.
4 Refer for specialist help as long-term HRT supervision is required to combat vulvovaginal atrophy and to restore libido.

Special points

1 A diagnosis of premature menopause often causes shock, disbelief, anger and regret. It requires special handling and adequate supervision of oestrogen replacement therapy.
2 Women with primary ovarian failure will occasionally recover and may conceive thereafter!

Hyperprolactinaemia
'Milk-like' substance can leak or be expressed by the patient from her nipple (galactorrhoea), but only occurs in less than 50% of cases.

Amenorrhoea — secondary

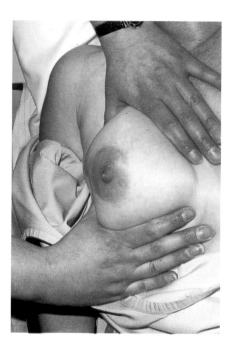

Fig 2.6 Expression of breast milk in hyperprolactinaemia.

1 The serum prolactin level may be mildly raised, and levels up to 1000 IU/l are not significant and are associated with stress and polycystic ovaries.

2 A level above 2000 IU/l suggests cranial pathology, and referral for magnetic resonance imaging (MRI) scan of the pituitary to diagnose a macro- or microadenoma is necessary.

3 Visual fields should also be checked.

4 Dopamine agonists such as Bromocriptine 2.5–7.5 mg daily or Cabergoline 0.5 mg twice weekly will bring the symptom under control, but may cause initial nausea and dizziness.

Amenorrhoea — secondary

5 When oestrogen levels rise during treatment, ovulation and menstruation will return and the oral contraceptive pill may be given for contraception.

6 Hyperprolactinaemia is idiopathic in 50% of cases.

7 Primary hypothyroidism is an uncommon cause, and a TSH level will make the diagnosis. Thyroxine replacement will correct the hyperprolactinaemia.

General management

1 Some patients require reassurance only that nothing sinister is causing the amenorrhoea.

2 Some are relieved not to have to cope with periods.

3 Barrier contraception should be used to prevent an unwanted pregnancy until ovulation resumes.

4 The oral contraceptive pill can also be used for cycle control, oestrogen therapy and endometrial protection.

5 Long-term effects of vaginal dryness and osteoporosis require HRT in women with oestrogen deficiency.

Oligomenorrhoea

The commonest cause of oligomenorrhoea (infrequent periods) is *polycystic ovarian disease*.

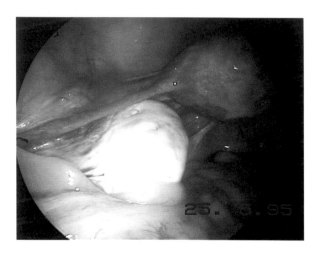

Fig 2.7 Large, pale, polycystic ovaries seen at laparoscopy.

Incidence
1–2% of young women present with oligomenorrhoea. They have erratic periods or regular, but infrequent, bleeds; in 90% of cases this is caused by polycystic ovaries.

Aetiology
This is a functional disorder of the ovary which may have a familial element.

Symptoms
1 Irregular cycles—6-weekly or a few times a year.
2 Hirsutism is present in 25% of cases due to raised androgen levels.

Oligomenorrhoea

3 Obesity with insulin resistance in some cases.
4 Infertility.
5 Acne on the face, chest and back.

Diagnosis (see p. 34)
1 Raised LH over 10 IU/l in 60% of cases.
2 Vaginal ultrasonography shows enlarged ovaries with increased stroma and the 'necklace' effect of peripheral unruptured follicles.
3 A progestogen challenge test (7 days of progestogen) will induce a bleed, as these women are well oestrogenised.

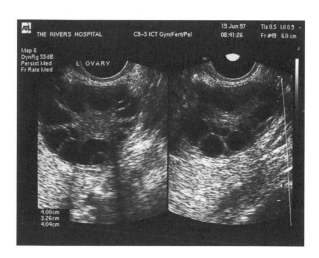

Fig 2.8 Scan of ovaries. 'Necklace effect'.

Management
1 Obese women should diet if possible, but many cannot achieve this goal.
2 A contraceptive pill, such as Dianette®, is useful for women requiring contraception.

Oligomenorrhoea

3 20% of women with this condition will ovulate and conceive naturally.

4 When fertility is required, ovulation induction with clomiphene citrate, 50 mg Day 2 to Day 6, can be tried after an induced bleed with a progestogen.

5 Clomiphene-resistant cases should be referred to a specialist clinic. Surgical procedures, such as ovarian multidiathermy, have led to ovulatory cycles.

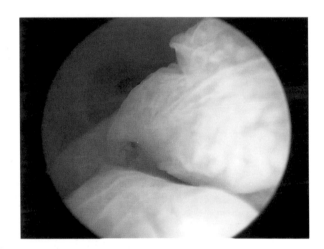

Fig 2.9 Endometrial hyperplasia. Note the thick, lush endometrium at hysteroscopy.

Special points

Women with this condition may develop endometrial hyperplasia and carcinoma, and regular withdrawal bleeds with the COCP or progestogens are advisable.

Dysmenorrhoea — primary

The commonest cause of menstrual problems in young women is *primary spasmodic dysmenorrhoea* (painful periods).

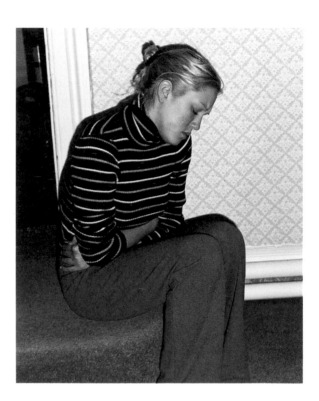

Fig 2.10 The teenager with dysmenorrhoea.

Incidence

1 80% of young women report dysmenorrhoea and 18% are severely affected.
2 Absenteeism from school and reduced performance in sport are commonplace.
3 Delayed child-bearing for career reasons lengthens the time span of this condition.

Dysmenorrhoea — primary

Aetiology

1 The release of circulating vasopressin causes myometrial hyperactivity and the secondary release of prostaglandins — $PGF_{2\alpha}$.

2 Child-bearing has an effect of decreasing dysmenorrhoea.

Symptoms

1 A build-up of crampy, colic-type pains, worse on the first and second days of flow.

2 Nausea and fainting may occur.

3 Premenstrual tension (PMT) may be associated.

4 Psychological overlay develops as the girl begins to 'dread her periods', and the mother is often involved in the care.

Management

1 History and examination to exclude pathology.

2 Reassurance and explanation of the pain and a positive attitude that it will improve with time.

3 A pelvic ultrasound examination can be reassuring that the pelvic organs are normal.

4 Advise use of:
   (a) simple analgesics, e.g. paracetamol;
   (b) COCP if contraception is required;
   (c) a non-steroidal anti-inflammatory drug (NSAID), e.g. mefenamic acid, 500 mg three times daily, or ketoprofen, 200 mg daily, during menstruation. The latter has a rapid uptake and action.

5 Keep a menstrual calendar and review every 2 months until pain is under control.

Special points

Some rare cases of primary dysmenorrhoea may be caused by genital tract abnormality, e.g. bicornate or bifid uterus, and will be diagnosed on ultrasonography and should be referred for specialist advice.

Dysmenorrhoea — primary

6 Very rarely a non-responder will require a laparoscopy to look for early endometriosis which can occur in teenage girls.

Dysmenorrhoea — secondary

The commonest symptom cited by the older woman in her request for a hysterectomy is *painful periods*.

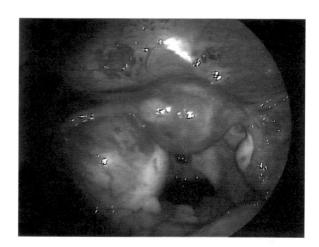

Fig 2.11 Severe endometriosis with peritoneal deposits, rectovaginal involvement. Left endometrioma.

Incidence
30% of women report menstrual pain, if asked, and self-medicate.

Aetiology
Prostaglandins appear to be the common mediator of crampy, uterine contractions in the case of the following.

Dysmenorrhoea—secondary

1 Endometriosis.
2 Fibroids.
3 An intrauterine contraceptive device (IUD).
4 Adenomyosis.
5 Pelvic inflammatory disease (PID).

Symptoms
1 Dull, pre- or postmenstrual ache.
2 Periods become heavy and 'clotty'.
3 Backache may be a significant symptom.
4 Deep dyspareunia.

Diagnosis
1 A history and pelvic examination to check for obvious pathology.
2 A pelvic ultrasound scan may suggest blood-filled cysts—endometrioma.
3 A menstrual calendar to chart the pain.

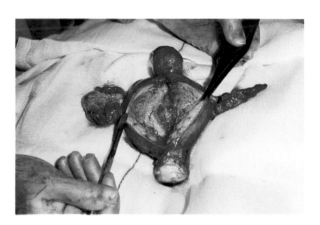

Fig 2.12 A hysterectomy specimen showing fibroids and adenomyosis.

Dysmenorrhoea — secondary

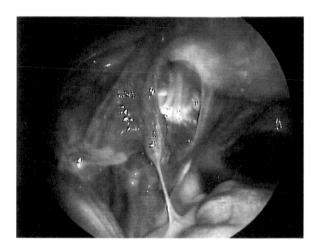

Fig 2.13 Pelvic inflammatory disease (PID).

Management

1 Remove IUD if present. Patients often demand this.

2 Therapeutic trial of NSAIDs, e.g. mefenamic acid or ibuprofen.

3 Refer for surgery if fibroids are present.

4 Refer for surgery if endometriosis or PID is suspected, or patient does not respond to a therapeutic trial of antibiotics and pain relief. Laparoscopy is the investigation of choice.

Dysmenorrhoea — secondary

Special points

Depressed and anxious women who are poly-symptomatic, with bowel and bladder dysfunction as well, are over-represented in this group of women. They use words such as 'horrendous' to describe pain and often have a normal uterus on pathological examination.

Treatment

Many women in this age group are not prepared to be inconvenienced by painful periods. Child-bearing is usually completed.

1 If pathology is diagnosed, a hysterectomy is often the best option to clear disease. Ovaries are usually preserved unless affected by disease.

2 The Mirena® intrauterine system (IUS) is being tried to control pain and excessive bleeding, and may be shown to have a role in the future.

Menorrhagia

The commonest cause of heavy periods is *fibroids*.

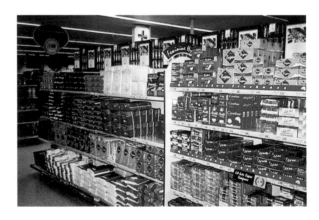

Fig 2.14 The commercial value of menstruation.

Menorrhagia

Incidence

1 30% of women in their reproductive years will report heavy periods to their GP.

2 The loss of over 80 ml of menstrual blood each month is regarded as heavy in research trials.

Aetiology

1 Fibroids are usually submucous—50% of cases.

2 Intrauterine polyps or IUD.

3 Endometriosis or adenomyosis.

4 Dysfunctional uterine bleeding (DUB).

Symptoms

1 The symptoms are very subjective and only 50% will actually have menorrhagia.

2 Heavy, short periods with clotting and flooding are also considered to be inconvenient and unacceptable by most women.

Management

1 Check for and treat anaemia if present. Surprisingly low haemoglobin (Hb) levels can be found.

2 Pelvic examination and cervical smear if indicated.

3 Pelvic ultrasound scan to detect fibroids and polyps.

4 Advise to keep a menstrual calendar for 3 months and record all symptoms and bleeds on it.

5 Obvious pathology will be detected on these investigations and appropriate referral will be

Special points

Rare causes of menorrhagia are clotting disorders, e.g. thrombocytopenic purpura and thyroid dysfunction.

Menorrhagia

made, but 50% of women have no detectable pathology and have DUB.

6 Early referral for laparoscopy if endometriosis is suspected.

7 Note length of history and degree of social inconvenience, e.g. absenteeism from work and disruption of life.

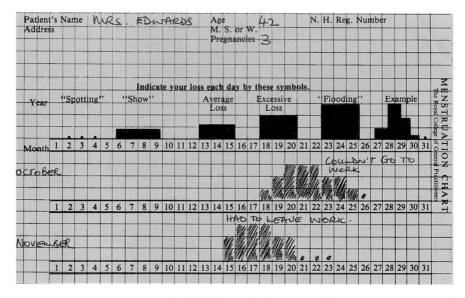

Fig 2.15 Menstrual calendar—useful record as many are returned with normal bleeding patterns. Can be obtained from the Royal College of General Practitioners.

Treatment of DUB

1 Oral contraceptive pill to suppress endometrial development.

2 NSAIDs, e.g. ibuprofen or mefenamic acid, during menstruation: very safe, reduce bleeding by 40% —may cause gastric irritation. Cost-

Menorrhagia

effective choice. Anti-prostaglandin agents.

3 Tranexamic acid, 1 g four times daily, Day 1 to Day 4 for six cycles. Can also produce gastro-intestinal symptoms. Expensive, but the most effective medical treatment. Anti-fibrinolytic agent.

Women over 40 years of age
Should be referred for hysteroscopy and endometrial biopsy as incidence of pelvic pathology is higher in this group.

Perimenopausal women
Short or irregular, anovulatory cycles can be managed with progestogen cyclically or HRT. *This is the only group in which progestogen is useful to control menorrhagia*, and high doses are recommended, e.g. norethisterone, 15 mg Day 5 to Day 26, but this is a short-term treatment.

Special points

Norethisterone is widely prescribed to control bleeding, but clinical trials have failed to show any advantage except in perimenopausal anovulatory women with erratic cycles. The levonorgestrel IUS is also effective in controlling DUB with reduction in blood loss of up to 97% after 12 months. It is a simple and effective alternative to surgery.

Indications for surgery
1 Pathology is present on scan or clinical examination or problem recurs.
2 Patient is dissatisfied with medical treatment.

Menorrhagia

3 Iron deficiency anaemia is the presenting symptom (often to medical clinics).
4 Patient is over 40 years of age.

Surgical management

Hysteroscopy and curettage or biopsy
1 Can be performed as an in- or out-patient and is carried out to detect pathology (Fig 2.16).
2 Polyps are very common and can be removed at diagnostic hysteroscopy under general anaesthetic by avulsion. They are usually benign (Fig 2.17).

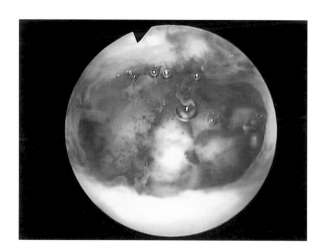

Fig 2.16 Normal endometrium with a uniform cavity.

Menorrhagia

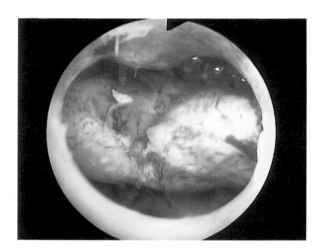

Fig 2.17 An intracavity polyp.

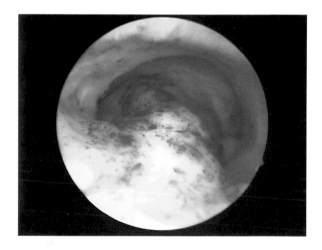

Fig 2.18 A submucous fibroid infiltrating the cavity.

3 Small, submucous fibroids can be identified and inspected but, if multiple or large, more definitive surgery is indicated, i.e. operative hysteroscopic resection or even hysterectomy (Fig 2.18).

Menorrhagia

4 Large plastic devices, e.g. Lippes Loop and Saf T Coils, can remain symptomless for years. If perimenopausal menorrhagia develops, removal may be difficult if threads are missing or the device is embedded in the uterine wall. Hysteroscopy confirms the location of the device and assists with removal (Fig 2.19).

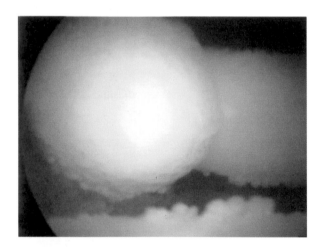

Fig 2.19 An embedded IUD.

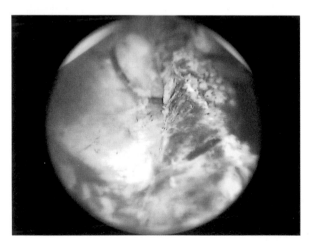

Fig 2.20 Resection of endometrium.

Menorrhagia

Transcervical resection of the endometrium (TCRE) (Fig 2.20)

1 Under general anaesthetic, the endometrium is cut or lasered away in deep strips until the myometrium is bare of endometrium.

2 Submucous fibroids and polyps may be dealt with by resection.

3 Day case or overnight stay. Quick recovery.

4 Good results with marked reduction in menstrual flow and amenorrhoea.

5 30% of cases of DUB are now treated by TCRE.

6 80% of patients are satisfied. One in six may require further surgery.

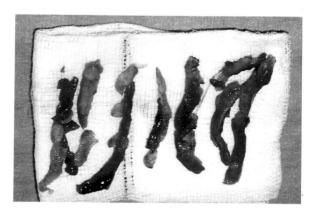

Fig 2.21 Strips of endometrium.

Menorrhagia

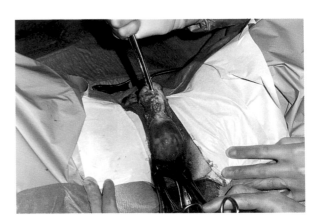

Fig 2.22 Simple vaginal hysterectomy.

Special points

The Mirena® IUS reduces blood loss dramatically, but is not licensed for the control of menorrhagia. Consider for women requiring contraception and with menorrhagia. Cost-effective choice of treatment.

Hysterectomy

65 000 hysterectomies are performed each year in the UK, of which 30 000 are for severe DUB.

1 For the older woman with prolapse, pathology or who wishes to obtain definitive relief of her symptoms.

2 Vaginal hysterectomy is a 'gold standard' operation with a good recovery time, but is not always possible if fibroids, adhesions or endometriosis are present.

3 Women are relieved to be released from monthly episodes of heavy blood loss and pelvic discomfort, and so are their partners.

4 'Painful, heavy periods' are the commonest cause for hysterectomy request in gynaecology clinics.

5 Menorrhagia results in a considerable loss of job attendance by women in the national workforce.

Menorrhagia

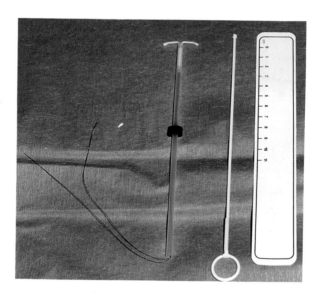

Fig 2.23 The Mirena® IUS.

Premenstrual tension

A common affliction experienced by 95% of normal women that causes upset and disruption of their lives.

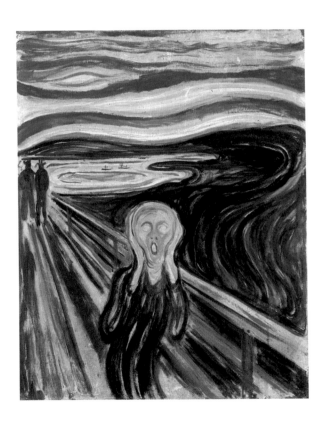

Fig 2.24 Edvard Munch *The Scream* 1893. Tempera on board. Copyright Munch Museum/Munch-Ellingsen Group/DACS 1998 (photograph © Munch Museum: Svein Andersen/Sidsel de Jong 1998).

Incidence
This syndrome of somatic and psychological symptoms causes 20% of normal, healthy women to seek help from their GP for emotional, behavioural and physical symptoms.

Aetiology
1 Only occurs with cyclical ovarian activity.

Premenstrual tension

2 In susceptible women, progesterone is a key factor.

3 Low levels of serotonin and β-endorphins have been cited.

Symptoms

1 Physical: headache, backache, bloating, weight gain, breast tenderness.

2 Emotional: depression, anxiety, irritability, fatigue, mood swings.

3 Behavioural: aggression, violence, food craving, poor concentration.

Diagnosis

1 'Self-diagnosis' on the patient's part.

2 There is no objective means for diagnosing or quantifying PMT.

Management

Mild to moderate cases

1 Exclude psychiatric condition. If 'menstrual distress' is severe and non-cyclical, may need psychiatric referral.

2 Advise a menstrual calendar for 2 months to chart symptoms which must be cyclical.

3 Sympathy, counselling and education on the physiological basis of the condition.

4 Symptom control:

  (a) simple analgesics for headache and pain;

  (b) breast pain (mastalgia): bromocriptine, 2.5 mg three times daily; Oil of Evening Primrose;

  (c) pelvic pain: danazol, 200 mg daily;

Premenstrual tension

(d) psychological symptoms and/or depression: fluoxetine, 20 mg daily;
(e) true cyclical water retention: spironolactone.

5 The majority of women only require reassurance and the above support.

6 Primary dysmenorrhoea associated with PMT should be treated with mefenamic acid or a COCP.

Severe cases

Suppress ovarian cycle with the following.

1 Oestrogen patches, 100–200 µg twice a week.

2 Oestrogen implants, 100 mg every 6 months. Women with an intact uterus will need endometrial control with either of the following.

3 Dydrogesterone, 10 mg daily for 14 days, for monthly bleeds.

4 Levonorgestrel IUS for suppression.

Intractable cases associated with severe domestic disruption

Refer for specialist gynaecological help.

1 Gonadotrophin-releasing hormone analogues, e.g. Zoladex®. Given monthly as subcutaneous pellet with 'add-back' oestrogen to prevent osteoporosis. Produces a 'medical oophorectomy'.

2 Surgery. This is the only 'cure' for PMT. A total hysterectomy with bilateral salpingo-oophorectomy and continuous oestrogen.

3 The following treatments have been used, but are unproven in clinical trials, and have a high placebo response:

(a) oral contraception;

Special points

1 Partners often accompany the patient and provide useful information on the severity of the symptoms and the impact on family life.

2 Some women on HRT will notice PMT symptoms, and a change to continuous combined therapy or tibolone is recommended.

Premenstrual tension

(b) dietary manipulation;
(c) vitamin B_6;
(d) Oil of Evening Primrose, except for mastalgia and in high doses: 4000 mg daily;
(e) diuretics.

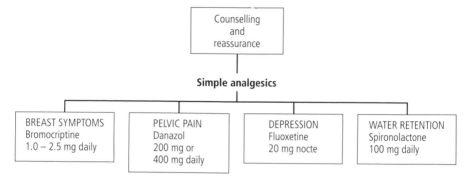

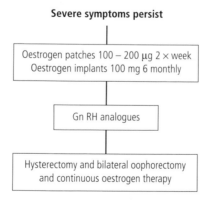

Fig 2.25 Flow chart of management.

Patient support services

1 National Association for Premenstrual Syndrome, PO Box 72, Sevenoaks, Kent, TN13 1XQ. Telephone: 01227 763 133.
2 PMS Help, PO Box 83, Hereford, HR4 8YQ.
3 Premenstrual Society, PO Box 429, Addleston, Surrey, KT15 1DZ.

3 Abnormal bleeding states

Intermenstrual bleeding

A common cause of consultation in the GP's surgery, but often resolved by the time of the specialist referral appointment!

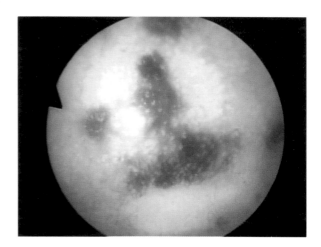

Fig 3.1 Hysteroscopic view of endometrium in patient with intermenstrual bleeding.

Incidence
1 Almost 80% of women in their reproductive years will experience an episode of intermenstrual bleeding.
2 It occurs between expected periods and can be light or heavy and of variable duration.

Aetiology
1 Breakthrough bleeding from contraceptive/hormonal use:
    (a) forgotten oral contraceptive pills;
    (b) progestogen-only pills taken erratically;
    (c) Depo-Provera injections in early months of treatment;
    (d) intrauterine contraceptive device (IUD) presence in the uterus;

Intermenstrual bleeding

(e) breakthrough bleeding on hormone replacement therapy (HRT).
2 Pelvic inflammatory disease (PID) with congestion.
3 Polyps in the cervix or uterus.
4 Submucous fibroids in the uterine cavity.
5 Endometriosis of the vaginal vault.

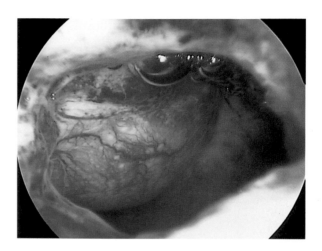

Fig 3.2 Submucous fibroid in the uterine cavity.

Special points

1 Young women reporting intermenstrual bleeding may have chlamydial cervicitis.
2 If these women are on the oral contraceptive pill, frequent changes of the pill will not help if chlamydial cervicitis is the cause.

Diagnosis

1 History of frequency and duration of symptoms.
2 Check that oral contraceptive pill or HRT has not been forgotten or missed.

Intermenstrual bleeding

3 Inspect the cervix for pathology and take a smear if one is due or if the cervix looks abnormal.

4 Take a chlamydial swab if appropriate.

5 Perform a bimanual examination to exclude upper genital tract tenderness and pathology of the vaginal vault.

6 Pelvic ultrasonography to check IUD location, fibroids and polyps.

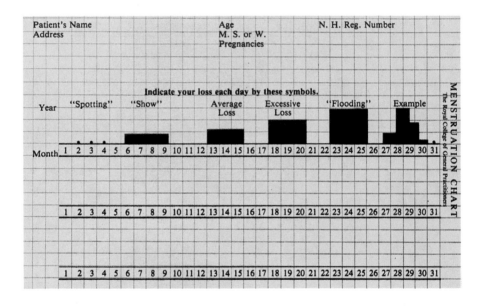

Fig 3.3 Menstrual calendar — can be useful.

Management

1 If pathology detected, refer for specialist advice.

2 Patient may request IUD removal.

3 Infection should be treated (see Chapter 4).

4 Hormonal contraception may need adjustment.

Intermenstrual bleeding

5 If no direct cause is found, ask the patient to keep a menstrual calendar for a few cycles. This can be very informative.

(a) If problems persist over three cycles, refer for specialist help, which may include hysteroscopy and curettage, especially if over 40 years of age.

(b) Many women will return a menstrual calendar that shows resolution of the complaint of intermenstrual bleeding without any treatment being needed.

Special points

Some women report that the intermenstrual bleeding followed a stressful episode in the family, e.g. death or illness, and this usually resolves spontaneously.

Postcoital bleeding

A common cause for alarm amongst women when bleeding follows sexual intercourse.

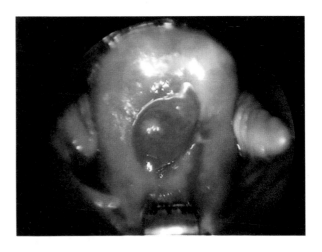

Fig 3.4 Polyp on cervix.

Postcoital bleeding

Incidence
1 About 10% of women will report this symptom after sexual intercourse or physical exercise, e.g. aerobics.
2 Bleeding may be brown streaking or fresh blood.

Aetiology
1 Cervical infection with:
    (a) *Chlamydia trachomatis*; or
    (b) chronic cervicitis of the transformation zone (an 'erosion').
2 Polyps:
    (a) endocervical polyps can bleed on impact;
    (b) uterine polyps can prolapse down the canal and cause congestive bleeding.

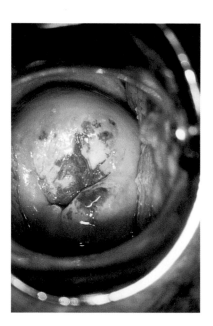

Fig 3.5 Early adenocarcinoma of the cervix. A 40-year-old woman presented with postcoital bleeding.

Postcoital bleeding

3 PID: chronic pelvic congestion may give rise to postcoital throbbing and slight bleeding.
4 Carcinoma of the cervix: a rare but significant presentation in the older woman and if glandular neoplasia is present up the endocervical canal.

Management
1 A thorough assessment of the lower genital tract with a Cusco speculum to view the vaginal walls and cervix for pathology.
2 Swabs for *Chlamydia* if there is a mucopurulent discharge from a red cervix, and appropriate antibiotic therapy.
3 A cervical smear if indicated or cervix looks abnormal.
4 Older women have more chance of pathology, and the exclusion of genital tract cancer is a priority. Refer early to the specialist clinic for:
    (a) pelvic ultrasonography;
    (b) endometrial sampling;
    (c) hysteroscopy with curettage and removal of intrauterine polyps;
    (d) diagnostic laparoscopy.

Postmenopausal bleeding

This is the most common presenting symptom of endometrial carcinoma.

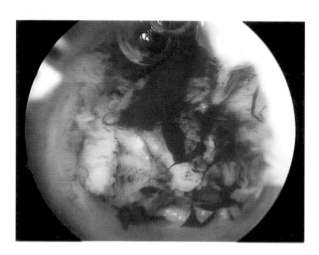

Fig 3.6 White, friable carcinoma in the uterus at hysteroscopy.

Incidence

1 A very common reason for consultation as many women in this age group are taking HRT and experience minor breakthrough bleeding.
2 Any woman who bleeds after the menopause has a 10–20% risk of having a genital cancer.

Aetiology

1 Breakthrough bleeding whilst on HRT, especially continuous combined therapy and tibolone.
2 Genital malignancy—may present as isolated or recurrent episodes. The most common mistake made in the diagnosis of cancer is the assumption that vaginal bleeding is due to atrophic vaginitis.

Postmenopausal bleeding

3 Many women have episodes that are 'unexplained'.
4 Atrophic vaginitis.
5 Polyps and fibroids.
6 Trauma.

Symptoms

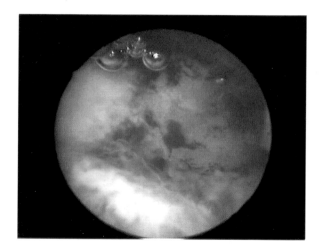

Fig 3.7 Hysteroscopic view of endometrium of patient who reported erratic bleeding on HRT.

1 Sudden vaginal bleeding occurring more than 6 months after menstruation has ceased.
2 Brown blood staining on underwear, intermittently.
3 The woman may consider any vaginal bleeding to be a 'period' and report: 'Periods come twice a month': 'Periods are all over the place'; 'I don't know when I am going to come on'. These bleeds are not periods and can be a symptom of serious gynaecological malignancy.

Postmenopausal bleeding

Problems with older women

1 Women are embarrassed to be examined while bleeding, and may cancel appointments with the GP or hospital clinic. Delay in examination can lead to delay in diagnosis of malignancy.
2 Bleeding may be ignored if it is light or intermittent in the hope that it will 'get better'.
3 Nursing an elderly or ailing husband may prevent a woman from seeking help for herself.
4 Postmenopausal bleeding is often blamed on domestic or social upsets.
5 Women often report the symptom when attending the doctor for another reason or when they are brought by a husband or daughter to whom they have confided.

Management

History
1 History of frequency, duration and amount of bleeding.
2 Relation to coitus, HRT usage and trauma.
3 Enquire about bladder function and haematuria.
4 Enquire about haemorrhoids and rectal bleeding.

Pelvic examination
Should never be delayed because patient is bleeding. Check for the following.
1 Urethral caruncle.
2 Vaginal nodules or growth.
3 Normal, atrophic cervix or vagina.
4 Normal, senile uterus and pelvic organs; ovaries not usually palpable.

Special points

1 Misinterpretation of this symptom is common in older women.
2 Repeated cancellations of appointments for 'bleeding' should arouse suspicion in receptionists and appointment clerks, and patients should be encouraged to attend despite bleeding.

Postmenopausal bleeding

5 Anaemia.

6 Rectal examination if patient will permit.

Investigations

1 A cervical smear is recommended.

2 Urine test for red blood cells.

3 A pelvic ultrasound and measurement of endometrial thickness can be arranged.

4 Refer early for specialist investigation which may be:

    (a) endometrial sampling and histology;

    (b) hysteroscopy and curettage;

    (c) endometrial scanning if not already performed.

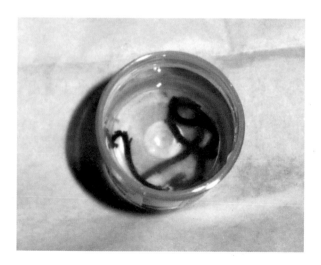

Fig 3.8 A core of aspirated endometrium for histology.

Diagnosis

The specialist clinic will advise on further treatment and follow-up. The following are the commonest diagnoses made at direct hysteroscopic examination of the uterus.

Postmenopausal bleeding

1 A normal, atrophic endometrium. A surprisingly common finding.

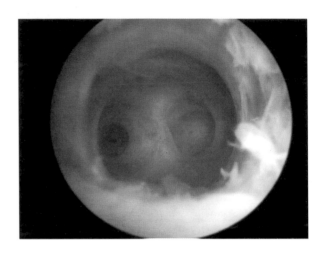

Fig 3.9 Normal, atrophic, postmenopausal uterus. Note fallopian tube ostia.

2 Endometrial carcinoma.

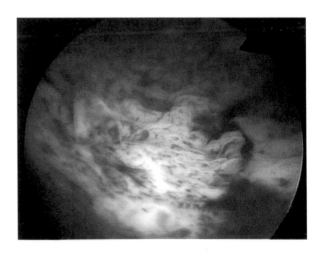

Fig 3.10 Endometrial carcinoma.

Postmenopausal bleeding

3 Endometrial polyps or fibroids.

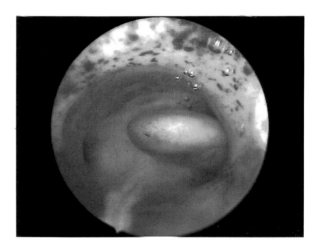

Fig 3.11 A fibroid polyp in a postmenopausal uterus.

Special points

1 Many cases investigated fail to show pathology.
2 Older women may confuse haematuria or rectal bleeding with vaginal bleeding.
3 Recurrent bleeders are more likely than 'one-off' bleeders to have carcinoma.
4 Atrophic vaginitis is easily treated with local oestrogen (oestriol pessaries), but may be masking the real culprit — a carcinoma further up the tract.

Postmenopausal bleeding

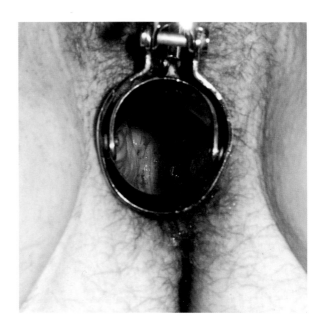

Fig 3.12 Atrophic vaginitis. Small, red pinpoints of haemorrhage due to epithelium thinning and oestrogen deficiency.

Adolescent menorrhagia

Anovulatory bleeding is common in adolescence.

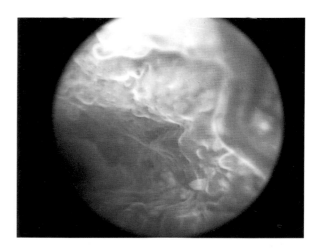

Fig 3.13 The lush endometrium of anovulatory hyperplasia in a 15-year-old girl.

Incidence
1 1–2 cases per year to the GP in girls aged 13–16 years.
2 50% of cycles are anovular in the first year after the menarche.

Aetiology
Anovulatory cycles with prolonged oestrogenic phase resulting in endometrial hyperplasia and flooding.

Symptoms
1 Prolonged, heavy bleeding throughout the month.
2 Severe haemorrhage necessitating admission to hospital and even transfusion.
3 Anaemia if severe.

Adolescent menorrhagia

4 Anxious mother.

5 Some will have continued menstrual problems throughout teenage years and may have polycystic ovaries diagnosed later.

Diagnosis
On history.

Management
1 Note weight, height and secondary sexual characteristics.

2 Enquire about absenteeism from school.

3 Reassure the girl and her mother that control can be achieved.

4 Check for anaemia with full blood count (FBC).

5 Instruct the girl to keep a menstrual calendar for 6 months.

6 If haemoglobin is less than 8 g, may need admission to hospital for transfusion.

7 Arrange a pelvic scan to ensure anatomical normality.

Special points

If the girl is anaemic, exclude a primary coagulation disorder.

Control of acute bleeding episode
1 Use the combined oral contraceptive pill (COCP) (30 µg ethinyloestradiol), one, four times daily, for 7 days. May cause nausea.
or:
2 Use medroxyprogesterone acetate, 30 mg daily for 10 days, or norethisterone, 5 mg daily for 7 days.

3 A withdrawal bleed will follow this therapy and, during this bleed, the COCP should be started and continued under supervision for 6 months.

Adolescent menorrhagia

4 If the COCP is not desired by the girl or her mother, intermittent progestogen—medroxy-progesterone acetate, 10 mg daily—can be given cyclically for 12 days each month to induce a bleed. Use for 6 months.

Control of heavy, regular periods
Mefenamic acid, 500 mg three times daily, during menses.

Resolution
Within 6 months, cycle control can be achieved and the treatment can be stopped so that spontaneous cycles can return and be assessed. The problem usually resolves. Supervision for a few years is required.

Special points

Some adolescents are sexually active, and these visits are an ideal time to address the issue of contraception.

Tamoxifen bleeding

A common cause of uterine bleeding in older women with breast cancer on tamoxifen therapy.

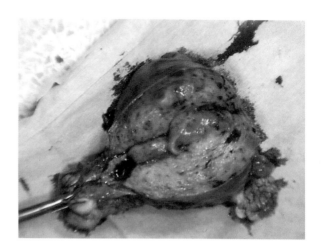

Fig 3.14 Hysterectomy specimen showing endometrial hyperplasia—patient on tamoxifen.

Incidence
Not yet quantified, but nearly all breast cancer patients will receive this drug as part of their therapy.

Aetiology
1 Tamoxifen promotes endometrial proliferation and both benign and malignant pathology.
2 It reduces the risk of relapse and death by 30% and that of developing a contralateral breast cancer by 40%.
3 Endometrial cancer is not common even in this group of women.

Diagnosis
1 By history and examination of the cervix.

Tamoxifen bleeding

2 Transvaginal ultrasound may show endometrial thickening or cystic spaces in the endometrium and proximal myometrium. Not specific enough to be used for screening asymptomatic women.

3 By hysteroscopy and curettage.

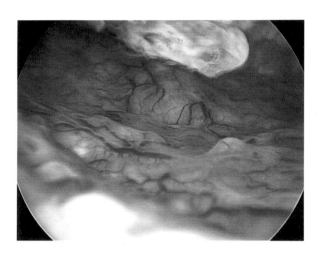

Fig 3.15 Note the vascularity and myometrial thickening in this 68-year-old woman on tamoxifen.

Treatment

1 Low-dose progestogens do not prevent endometrial hyperplasia and, by extension, a levonorgestrel intrauterine system (IUS) may not be effective.

2 Repeated bleeds induce great anxiety in women who are already dealing with cancer of the breast.

3 Operative procedures rather than observation may be preferred, and could be transcervical resection of the endometrium (TCRE) or hysterectomy, especially if myometrial pathology is also present.

Endometrial sampling

A commonly used technique in the out-patient setting to obtain endometrial tissue for assessment.

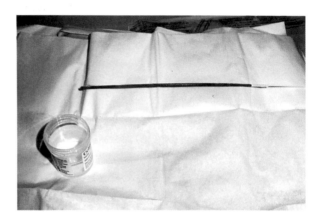

Fig 3.16 The Pipelle suction device aspirates endometrium for histology.

Devices used, e.g. Pipelle, Gynocheck
1 They are used:
    (a) in out-patient surgery and well tolerated;
    (b) without the need for anaesthesia;
    (c) to aspirate a core of endometrial tissue.
2 Advantages:
    (a) quick and usually easy technique;
    (b) avoids admission and general anaesthesia;
    (c) good correlation with subsequent pathology;
    (d) provides a good specimen.
3 Disadvantages:
    (a) difficulty with insertion in post-menopausal women with cervical stenosis;
    (b) can be painful in some cases;
    (c) lack of tissue aspirate does not exclude

Endometrial sampling

serious disease; sensitivity of 73% when used alone;

(d) the cervix may need to be grasped with a tenaculum to provide counterpressure; this increases pain and bleeding;

(e) advise risk of postaspiration bleeding and cramping.

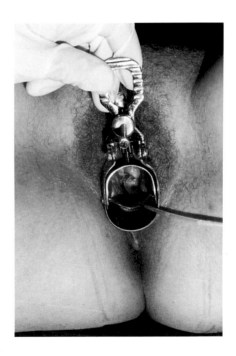

Fig 3.17 Pipelle in uterus aspirating tissue.

Indications

Assessment of the endometrium in the following.

1 Breakthrough bleeding on HRT and contraceptives.

2 Infertility cases for endometrial assessment.

3 Postmenopausal bleeding.

Endometrial sampling

4 Menorrhagia in women over 40 years of age.
5 Heavy perimenopausal bleeding—endometrial carcinoma can occur premenopause.
6 Any bizarre, erratic or abnormal bleeding pattern in women over 40 years of age.
7 Used in combination with transvaginal ultrasound or diagnostic hysteroscopy, it can detect 90% of endometrial disease.

Hysteroscopy

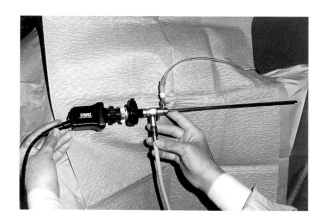

Fig 3.18 The hysteroscope.

1 Hysteroscopy and curettage is now considered to be the 'gold standard' for endometrial assessment and has replaced dilation and curettage (D & C).
2 Combined with transvaginal ultrasonography and biopsy, almost 90% of endometrial pathology can be diagnosed.

Hysteroscopy

3 Small-diameter telescopes (2.5 mm) are available for out-patient assessment without an anaesthetic and using gas or saline as a distension medium. The cervix does not need to be dilated, local anaesthetic is unnecessary in 70% of cases and the procedure is well tolerated.

4 For anxious patients or those who cannot tolerate the procedure, a general anaesthetic as a day case is used. A larger diameter telescope can be passed through the dilated cervix and an endoscopic camera allows magnification on a video monitor. Excellent views of the cavity and diagnoses of fibroids, polyps and other endometrial pathologies can be obtained. Photographs can be taken for permanent records and for patient information.

4 Pelvic infection and sexually transmitted disease

Pelvic inflammatory disease (PID)

One of the commonest referrals to the emergency gynaecology service in hospital is the young woman with suspected PID.

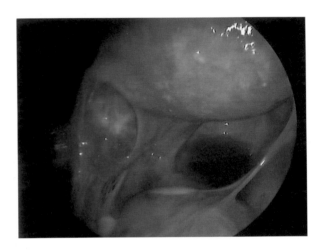

Fig 4.1 A view of the pelvis after infection—adhesions and tubal blockage.

Incidence
1 In general practice, 13 out of 1000 women per year will have PID diagnosed.
2 Only 10% of these will be admitted to hospital.

Aetiology
1 *Chlamydia trachomatis*—responsible for 50% of cases.
2 *Neisseria gonorrhoeae*—declining in importance.
3 Anaerobes, e.g. *Mycoplasma hominis*, have an unclear role.

Pelvic inflammatory disease (PID)

Symptoms
1 Vaginal discharge.
2 Pelvic pain and tenderness.
3 Dyspareunia.
4 Dysuria.
5 Cervical excitation.
6 Fever.
7 Pelvic mass.
8 Women may not be 'ill' with the infection.

Diagnosis
1 History of lower abdominal pain and, possibly, vaginal discharge.
2 Pelvic tenderness on bimanual examination and with cervical excitation.
3 Take swabs from the urethra, cervix and posterior vaginal fornix for culture and sensitivity prior to treatment and for Gram stains.
4 An air-dried smear of vaginal secretion on a slide should be sent for a Gram stain.
5 Cervical swab for chlamydia antigen — enzyme-linked immunosorbent assay (ELISA).
6 Refer to genitourinary medicine (GUM) clinic if patient will agree or to hospital if pyrexial and 'toxic'.

Treatment
Antibiotic therapy must be effective against chlamydia, gonorrhoea and the anaerobes of bacterial vaginosis. Treatment should be commenced on presentation and symptoms.
1 Pyrexial, ill patients usually in hospital: cefoxitin, 2 g intravenously every 6 h for 48–72 h, plus

Special points
1 Ectopic pregnancy is more frequent in women with past episodes of PID and may even mimic it at presentation.
2 If there is any doubt about the diagnosis, refer to gynaecology service, where laparoscopy may be indicated to exclude ectopic pregnancy and confirm the diagnosis of infection.

Pelvic inflammatory disease (PID)

doxycycline, 100 mg orally twice daily for 14 days.

2 Out-patients: ofloxacin, 400 mg orally twice daily, plus clindamycin, 450 mg orally four times daily, or metronidazole, 400 mg orally twice daily. All for 14 days.

3 Women undergoing induced abortion could have metronidazole, 1 g rectally at operation, plus doxycycline, 100 mg orally twice daily for 7 days.

4 Women under 35 years of age undergoing intrauterine contraceptive device (IUD) insertion, laparoscopy for infertility investigation or endometrial sampling could have metronidazole, 1 g rectally, and doxycycline, 100 mg orally twice daily for 7 days.

Sexual partners of women with PID

1 Partners are usually infected and may have no symptoms.

2 Contact tracing and screening in GUM clinics are very important.

3 Sexual partners can be treated empirically with the same regimen if unwilling to undergo screening.

4 Microbiological proof of infection may be difficult to obtain, and therefore treatment should be on symptoms and include *both* partners.

Long-term sequelae

1 Chronic pelvic pain in 50% of PID patients.

2 Infertility in 30% of PID patients.

3 Ectopic pregnancy.

Pelvic inflammatory disease (PID)

4 Frequent hospital admissions.
5 In long-standing cases, early recourse to hysterectomy to relieve symptoms.

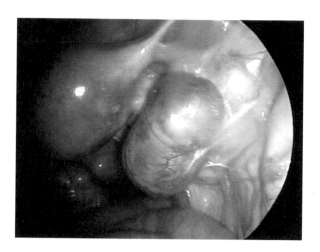

Fig 4.2 Chronic pelvic pain and infertility from hydrosalpinges.

Sexually transmitted disease (STD)

The commonest STD in the world is *chlamydia*.

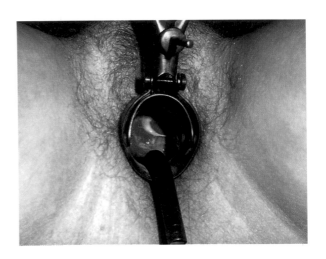

Fig 4.3 Mucopurulent discharge from a red cervix.

Incidence
1 Up to 12% of women under 25 years of age become infected.
2 Infections are often asymptomatic and go untreated.
3 Many women present as a consequence of symptoms in their partner.

Aetiology
Chlamydia trachomatis harboured in the endocervical canal.

Symptoms
1 75% of women have no symptoms.
2 Mucopurulent vaginal discharge.
3 Dysuria.

Sexually transmitted disease (STD)

4 Postcoital bleeding.
5 Intermenstrual bleeding.
6 Dyspareunia and pelvic pain.

Diagnosis
This is an intracellular organism, and it can be difficult to obtain an adequate tissue sample from the endocervix for diagnosis.
1 Endocervical swab: current techniques for diagnosing chlamydia are not ideal. Enzyme immunoassays are widely used in general practice, but only have sensitivities of 60–80% when compared with optimal methods, but are cost-effective. Deoxyribonucleic acid (DNA) amplification technique on first-void urine specimens is the most effective and acceptable way to screen and is under review.
2 High degree of suspicion.
3 Red, inflamed cervix on speculum examination.

Management
1 Refer to GUM clinic, if possible, to screen for concomitant sexual infection. (GP referral rate is only 15–30%.)
2 Partners must be included as 80% will be infected.

Patients to target for screening
1 Referrals for pregnancy termination—8% incidence.
2 Women attending for emergency contraception.

Sexually transmitted disease (STD)

3 Women attending GUM clinics.
4 Women attending emergency gynaecological services with vaginal discharge and pelvic pain.
5 Consider in patients attending for IUD insertion as this may predispose to upper tract infection.

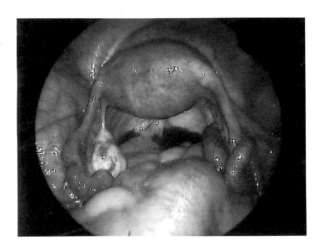

Fig 4.4 Hydrosalpinx and tubal blockage after pregnancy termination 1 year previously.

Treatment
1 Doxycycline, 100 mg twice daily for 7 days.
2 In complicated infections, where poor compliance on therapy may occur, azithromycin, 1 g single oral dose.
3 Erythromycin, 500 mg four times daily for 7 days, in pregnant or lactating women.
4 Ofloxacin, 400 mg daily for 5 days. A good choice as bactericidal.

Sexually transmitted disease (STD)

Long-term sequelae

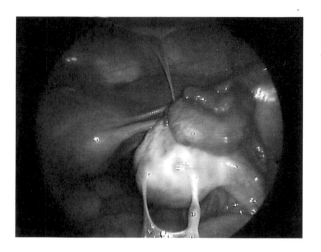

Fig 4.5 Blocked tube and adhesions.

1 Chlamydia can persist for long periods if untreated.

2 30% of inadequately treated women will develop PID which can cause:

    (a) infertility;

    (b) ectopic pregnancy;

    (c) chronic pelvic pain;

    (d) dyspareunia.

3 Chlamydia has been associated with obstetric problems of intrauterine growth retardation and prematurity.

Sexually transmitted disease (STD)

Special points

1 Any young woman with any of the following symptoms should be screened and treated for chlamydia if appropriate:

   (a) postcoital bleeding;

   (b) intermenstrual bleeding;

   (c) breakthrough bleeding on the oral contraceptive pill.

2 Remember it is the young 'pill taker' who is most at risk of contracting the infection.

5 Pelvic pain

Acute pelvic pain

Pelvic inflammatory disease (PID)

The commonest cause of the onset of acute pelvic pain in young women is pelvic inflammatory disease (PID), see Chapter 4 for aetiology, diagnosis and management.

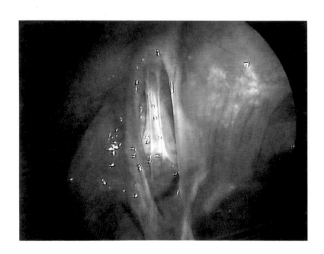

Fig 5.1 Note the chlamydial adhesions around left ovary.

Summary of key points in diagnosis and management

1 Bilateral pelvic pain and vaginal discharge.

2 Postcoital pain and bleeding.

3 Needs antibiotic therapy and contact tracing.

4 May become chronic pain with serious long term sequelae.

5 Refer to genitourinary medicine (GUM) clinic if possible before initial treatment is given so that swabs can be taken, but, if severe attack, commence antibiotics immediately.

6 Refer after treatment for follow-up to GUM clinic if urgent therapy was indicated. This allows treatment of partner.

Special points

Bactericidal drugs such as Ofloxacin are preferred to bacteriostatic drugs.

Acute pelvic pain

Urinary tract infection (UTI)

Another common cause of the onset of acute pelvic pain in young women.

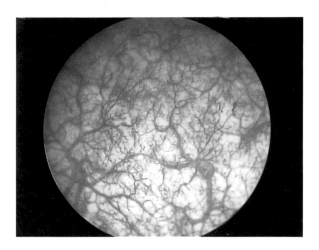

Fig 5.2 The inflamed urothelium at cystoscopy.

Symptoms
1 Sudden onset of central bladder pain.
2 Dysuria and frequency.
3 Can have frank haematuria.
4 Often pyrexial with smelly, cloudy urine.

Diagnosis
1 Usually self-diagnosed.
2 Midstream urine (MSU) sample should be sent to laboratory for confirmation.

Treatment
1 Needs chemotherapeutic agents, such as:
    (a) trimethoprim, 200 mg twice daily for 5 days;
    (b) nitrofurantoin, 50 mg four times daily for 7 days;

Acute pelvic pain

(c) norfloxacin, 400 mg twice daily for 3 days;
(d) Augmentin®, 375 mg three times daily for 4 days.

2 Recurrent attacks need referral for renal tract assessment by imaging and endoscopy.

3 See Chapter 10 for further information.

Ectopic pregnancy

A very important cause of pelvic pain in young women.

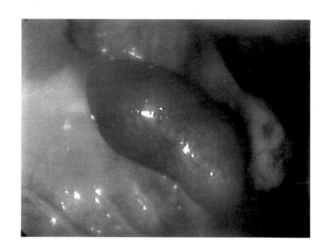

Fig 5.3 The extrauterine implantation of the gestation sac usually in the fallopian tube.

Incidence

1 Dramatic increase in incidence, and many referrals by GPs to accident and emergency departments to exclude ectopic pregnancy. About 10 000 cases a year in the UK.

2 25–50% of suspected cases are subsequently discharged as diagnosis not confirmed.

Aetiology

1 Clinical or subclinical tubal damage from

Acute pelvic pain

chlamydial infection resulting in inability of tubal ciliated epithelium to transport blastocyst to the uterine cavity.
2 Incomplete blockage of tube by fibrosis.
3 Assisted reproduction and reconstructive surgery.

Symptoms
1 Patient usually aware of early pregnancy status with nausea, sore breasts, etc.
2 Sharp pain in one or other iliac fossa.
3 Last period may not have been missed, but could be lighter or atypical.
4 Brownish, intermittent vaginal bleeding.
5 Delay in diagnosis will lead to tubal rupture with intraperitoneal haemorrhage. This may be acute with collapse and shock due to the haemoperitoneum, or may become chronic with the development of a pelvic mass and old 'walled-off' bleeding and adhesions.

Cautionary note — 'A Great Masquerader'
Delay in diagnosis is a common cause for complaint and litigation and the GP is often involved. Can be very difficult to diagnose and will catch the unwary out frequently! Women are occasionally discharged from hospital after negative investigation, only to be readmitted a week later with haemoperitoneum.

Diagnosis
1 Refer on clinical suspicion: pain, bleeding and amenorrhoea.
2 Early transvaginal ultrasound scan will usually show the gestation sac in the tube or

Special points
Any erratic vaginal bleeding and pelvic pain in a woman in her reproductive years should alert the clinician to consider a diagnosis of ectopic pregnancy.

Acute pelvic pain

indicate a complex mass in either adnexa. Uterine cavity will be empty on scan.

3 Human chorionic gonadotrophin (HCG) assay, now performed almost routinely in accident and emergency departments, will confirm pregnancy and, combined with the above, will alert the clinician to the possibility of an ectopic.

4 Diagnostic laparoscopy undertaken under general anaesthetic will confirm the swollen tube, often with a bluish appearance, and there may be fimbrial bleeding.

5 With early suspicion, the diagnosis can be achieved in most cases before tubal rupture.

6 One in five women referred with a suspected ectopic pregnancy undergo laparoscopy and is found to be normal.

7 If tubal rupture has occurred, there will be frank blood in the pelvis. Immediate laparotomy is performed.

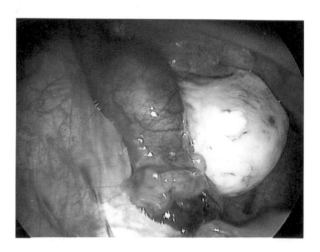

Fig 5.4 Gestation sac starting to abort and bleed through fimbrial end.

Acute pelvic pain

Treatment

Spontaneous tubal abortion
Ten per cent of women can successfully abort or resorb the conceptus from the tube if kept *under strict medical supervision* and HCG levels are monitored frequently. Few, however, would wish this course of action.

Medical management
1 Methotrexate can be used systemically, or injected into the tube to cause tubal abortion for early cases under 2 cm in tubal diameter.
2 Not routine unless patient wishes to avoid tubal surgery, but good results of subsequent tubal patency (90%). Low recurrence rate of repeat ectopic (12%) and intrauterine pregnancy rate of 85%.

Surgery
1 Laparoscopy: if the tube is unruptured at diagnostic laparoscopy.
   (a) The tube can be opened, the gestation sac sucked out and the tube left to heal spontaneously — salpingostomy. A tubal patency rate of 80% has been reported afterwards, but the recurrent ectopic pregnancy rate is 22% and the intrauterine pregnancy rate is 60%.
   (b) The affected segment of the tube can be excised with diathermy and removed, or the whole tube if obviously damaged can be removed — salpingectomy. The subsequent intrauterine pregnancy rate is 40%.
   (c) Laparoscopic surgery demands good technical expertise and haemostasis. Patients

Acute pelvic pain

can be discharged the next day with an expectation of rapid recovery and a good cosmetic result.

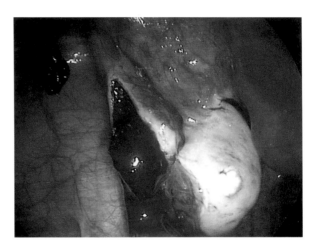

Fig 5.5 Laparoscopic salpingostomy to remove the gestation sac.

2 Laparotomy: if the tube has ruptured or the gestation sac is large, the open method is preferred.

(a) It is safe, quick and haemostasis is rapidly achieved.

(b) Many cases of ectopic pregnancy are handled at night by subconsultant grade staff and safety is paramount. Death from haemorrhagic shock is still reported in *Confidential Enquiries into Maternal Deaths in the United Kingdom* as accounting for 9.1% of all deaths in the period under study 1994–96.

Screening
Women who should be screened early for ectopic pregnancy by ultrasound in the next pregnancy include the following.

Acute pelvic pain

1 Those who have had a previous ectopic pregnancy. Risk increased tenfold.

2 Those who have had a previous episode of severe PID requiring admission to hospital. Risk increased fourfold.

3 Intrauterine contraceptive device (IUD) wearers with symptoms of early pregnancy.

4 Women with two or more previous episodes of PID managed by their GP.

5 Women who have undergone tubal reanastomosis or tubal sterilisation. Risk increased 4.5-fold.

6 Women with a history of severe appendicitis or previous peritonitis from whatever cause.

7 Women with a history of infection after abortion, delivery or hysterosalpingogram (HSG).

8 *Early screening* will lead to *early diagnosis* which will lead to *early surgical evaluation* and preservation of the tube with an increased chance of subsequent fertility.

Fertility after ectopic pregnancy

1 About 15% of patients will develop a recurrent ectopic pregnancy in subsequent pregnancies.

2 The results after laparoscopic surgery are not yet available.

3 Contraception after an ectopic pregnancy can safely be provided with a copper IUD or Mirena® intrauterine system (IUS), as well as the combined oral contraceptive pill (COCP).

Special points

'Have a high index of suspicion and investigate properly': quoted by Catherine E. James, Medicolegal Adviser, Medical Defence Union.

Cyclical pelvic pain

The commonest cause of cyclical pelvic pain in young women is spasmodic dysmenorrhoea (see Chapter 2); in women in their reproductive years is endometriosis and in older women is adenomyosis.

Endometriosis

Tissue deposits resembling endometrium located outside the uterus on the tubes, ovaries, ligaments and peritoneum.

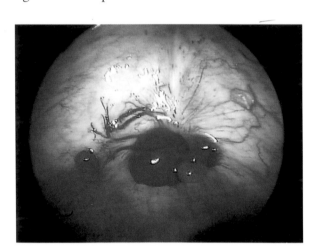

Fig 5.6 Active deposit of endometriosis on peritoneum.

Incidence
1 Unknown, as lesions often found in 10% of non-symptomatic women, but rising to 40% in infertile women.
2 Minor degrees of endometriosis are common and of no clinical significance.

Aetiology
1 The exact aetiology and pathogenesis of the condition remain unclear.

Cyclical pelvic pain

2 The tissue is oestrogen responsive and monthly menstrual soiling of the peritoneal cavity occurs. Retrograde menstrual flow is probably implicated.

3 Peritoneal, ovarian and rectovaginal septum endometriosis probably have different aetiological origins and are thought to be different diseases.

Classical symptoms

1 Deep dyspareunia.

2 Cyclical pelvic pain.

3 Central abdominal pain and backache.

4 Menorrhagia.

5 Dysmenorrhoea—secondary congestive.

Diagnosis

1 Clinical suspicion on the part of the GP.

2 Tender, fixed, retroverted uterus on bimanual palpation.

3 Tender nodules may be felt around uterine ligaments or in vaginal vault.

4 Pelvic scan may show enlarged ovaries with endometriomas 'chocolate cysts'.

5 Laparoscopy is essential to confirm the diagnosis and to assess the extent of the disease.

Special points

Pelvic pain that persists for longer than 6 months should be investigated by diagnostic laparoscopy.

Cyclical pelvic pain

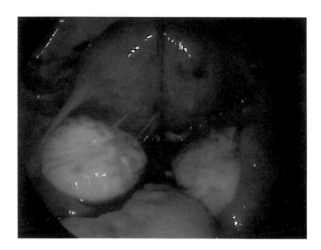

Fig 5.7 Endometriosis seen at laparoscopy.

Consequences of endometriosis to the patient
1 May be a symptomless incidental finding of no consequence.
2 Subfertility.
3 Progressive fibrosis and scarring of pelvic organs with adherence to each other and obliteration of the pouch of Douglas.
4 Painful defaecation if rectovaginal septum infiltrative disease is present.
5 Development of 'enlarged chocolate cysts' on ovaries.
6 Some women may be reduced to being 'pelvic cripples'.

Treatment

Asymptomatic women
1 Do not need therapy.
2 Condition recedes after menopause.

Cyclical pelvic pain

Mild disease

1 Medical therapy can be tried if symptoms are present and inconvenient.

 (a) Continuous oral progestogen: medroxy-progesterone acetate, 30 mg daily, or dydro-gesterone, 30 mg daily.

 (b) Synthetic androgen: danazol, 400 mg daily continuously.

 (c) Gonadotrophin releasing hormone (GnRH) analogues: Zoladex®, 3.6 mg depot monthly for 4–6 months.

 (d) Continuous COCP.

2 30–60% pregnancy rate can be achieved after treatment with danazol and GnRH analogues.

Special points

1 Danazol and Zoladex® treatment is associated with weight gain, flushing and acne.

2 Zoladex® may also result in bone loss after 6 months, and 'add-back oestrogen' may be prescribed.

3 Patients may not wish to experience these symptoms, in which case surgical therapy is preferred.

Moderate to severe disease

1 Surgical therapy by laparotomy or laparoscopy. Aim is to clear endometriomas of ovaries and adhesiolysis, to restore the mobility of tubes and ovaries and to ablate deposits of disease in the peritoneum. Electrical diathermy or laser may be used.

2 40–60% pregnancy rate can be achieved after this type of treatment.

Cyclical pelvic pain

3 The object of treatment is to relieve pelvic pain and restore fertility.

4 Patients who desire a pregnancy usually opt for surgical treatment as medical therapy depresses fertility for almost a year.

5 Some women who fail to conceive after surgery are best referred for assisted conception, e.g. gamete intrafallopian transfer (GIFT) or *in vitro* fertilisation (IVF).

6 After child-bearing, some patients are better off being offered a hysterectomy and removal of both ovaries, and hormone replacement therapy (HRT) thereafter with a continuous combined formulation.

7 Retention of the ovaries can allow pain to persist — 'remnant ovary syndrome'.

8 Surgery for advanced endometriosis is hazardous.

9 HRT does not necessarily result in symptom recurrence.

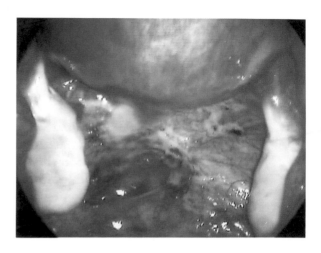

Fig 5.8 Pouch of Douglas disease treated by bipolar diathermy. Note scarring and 'pocketing' in the peritoneal pouch.

Cyclical pelvic pain

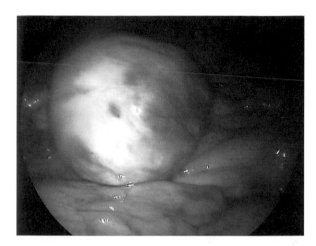

Fig 5.9 An endometrioma.

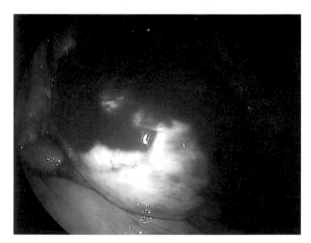

Fig 5.10 Note chocolate fluid — old blood in this cyst.

Patient advice
Living with Endometriosis — A Patient's Guide to the Disease and its Treatment — Zeneca.

Cyclical pelvic pain

Adenomyosis

A common cause of cyclical pelvic pain in older women.

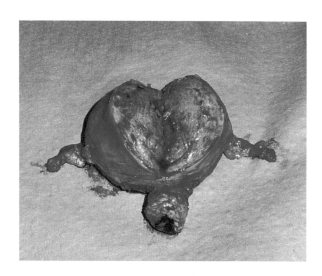

Fig 5.11 The bulky uterus at hysterectomy. Note thickened walls.

Incidence
Reported by pathologists on histology of 40% of perimenopausal women who have undergone hysterectomy.

Aetiology
Unknown factors allow endometrial glands to creep into myometrial layers of uterus.

Symptoms
1 Painful periods, but only 40% of cases will have heavy periods.
2 Dull, low pelvic ache for many days post-menstrually.
3 Dyspareunia and often premenstrual tension (PMT) and congestion.

Cyclical pelvic pain

Diagnosis
1 Bulky, tender uterus.
2 Ultrasound not helpful unless cystic spaces seen in myometrium—accumulations of blood.
3 Usually retrospective histological diagnosis.
4 A laparoscopy is often recommended to exclude other pathology.

Treatment
1 Responds poorly to medical treatment.
2 Recommend hysterectomy if suspected and child-bearing complete. Relief from the misery of painful, heavy periods each month is welcomed.

Special points

1 Because of the difficulty with the diagnosis clinically, many women with adenomyosis and heavy periods are offered a resection of the endometrium.
2 After this, deeply situated glands can regrow and symptoms may recur, with a failure of the operative procedure to control the symptoms.

Chronic pelvic pain

A common cause for referral to the gynaecology clinic. A difficult symptom complex to sort out.

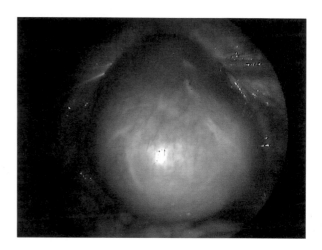

Fig 5.12 Large fibroid causing low pelvic pain/backache.

Incidence
Up to one-third of new referrals to out-patients are for chronic pelvic pain.

Aetiology
1 Pathological conditions such as endometriosis, infection and pelvic masses, e.g. fibroids.
2 Genital prolapse.
3 Irritable bowel syndrome.
4 Chronic pelvic congestion.
5 Depression, anxiety.
6 Vulvodynia.

Chronic pelvic pain

Diagnosis and management of the causes of chronic pelvic pain usually in older women

Vulvodynia
1 The development of an unremitting, burning, vaginal pain usually in older women with no obvious aetiological cause.
2 Severe upset to life occurs with multiple therapies prescribed.
3 Usually depressed and overwhelmed by the intense pain.
4 Reassurance that the condition is well known.
5 Patients need constant support and advice.
6 Tricyclic antidepressants at low dose may work: amitriptyline, 25 mg *nocte*.
7 No known cure, and prognosis for the resolution of symptoms cannot be given.
8 One of the most difficult conditions to treat and manage.
9 Refer to specialist vulval clinic.

Pelvic tumours
1 Fibroids and ovarian cysts may cause pressure symptoms and discomfort.
2 A pelvic ultrasound scan will confirm their presence.
3 Refer for surgical assessment.
4 In older women, signs of malignancy should be sought — lymphadenopathy, swollen legs or abdomen, anaemia.

Irritable bowel syndrome
1 Usually left iliac fossa (LIF) pain more than once a month and relief with defaecation.

Chronic pelvic pain

2 Abdominal distension with episodes of diarrhoea alternating with constipation.
3 May respond to fibre bulking agent and antispasmodics, e.g. mebeverine.

Genital prolapse
1 A deep, dragging, pelvic pain worse towards the end of the day and usually associated with obvious tissue prolapse at introitus.
2 Will require referral for surgical assessment.

Diagnosis and management of the causes of chronic pelvic pain in younger women

Psychosomatic pelvic pain
1 There is a group of women in whom depression, introspection and relationship difficulties are common and who present with pelvic pain.
2 In this group, there is a high incidence of childhood sexual abuse and adult abusive relationships.
3 A careful and sensitive history is essential at the first consultation, including sexual and social problems.
4 Counselling is the mainstay of management.

Special points

1 Patients often treated with repeated courses of antibiotics with variable response.
2 Negative laparoscopy or minor pathology only.
3 Patients become demoralised with low self-esteem.

Chronic pelvic pain

Chronic pelvic congestion or pelvic pain syndrome

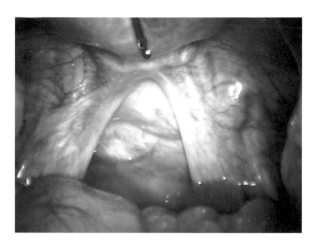

Fig 5.13 Chronic venous congestion of the pelvic veins.

1 Venous congestion with deep dyspareunia and postcoital aching.
2 Worse premenstrually and on prolonged standing.
3 High incidence of stress and anxiety and resultant sexual problems.
4 Pain is non-specific in site and often radiates down the legs.
5 Pelvic ultrasound scan may show enlarged ovaries and dilated pelvic veins may be seen.
6 Diagnostic laparoscopy indicated to assess pelvis and exclude endometriosis.
7 Treated with high-dose Provera®, 50 mg daily.
8 Counselling and stress reduction techniques especially for depression and mood disorder.

Special points

Ultrasound is more useful than laparoscopy unless endometriosis is suspected.

History
1 It is important to watch patient carefully

Chronic pelvic pain

during consultation. She may be depressed, defensive or even hostile.

2 Bowel and bladder function must be ascertained.

3 Sexual problems or unhappy memories can be gently elicited.

4 Past psychiatric illness can be important.

Examination

In all cases of chronic pelvic pain, examination must include the following.

1 Abdominal palpation for masses, ascites.

2 Pelvic examination.

3 Rectal check for masses or malignancy.

Investigations

1 Pelvic scan to exclude pathology.

2 Refer for diagnostic laparoscopy if pain has been present for 6 months or more in young women. A negative laparoscopy can be reassuring and helpful.

3 An MSU sample for infection is mandatory.

4 Pelvic venography — specialist clinic will arrange.

5 Chlamydial swab — immunofluorescence may be useful.

Special points

1 Radical surgery may have to be considered for severely disabled chronic cases, and would be a hysterectomy and bilateral salpingo-oophorectomy.

2 Despite this, the patient may continue to present to her GP with abnormal pain and backache.

Dyspareunia

A common condition in both young and old with somatic and psychological elements. The diagnosis and management of individual conditions are dealt with in the appropriate chapters.

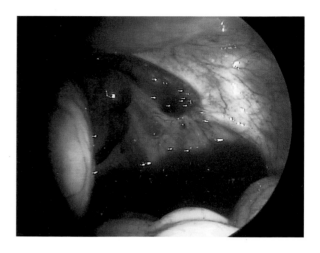

Fig 5.14 Deep, infiltrative endometriosis in pouch of Douglas.

Young women — superficial dyspareunia
1 Infection — *Candida* and bacterial vaginosis.
2 Scars — episiotomy scar after delivery.
3 Hormonal — breast-feeding mothers, vaginal dryness.
4 Vaginismus — fear of penetration, non-consummation of marriage.
5 Psychosexual — fear of sexually transmitted disease (STD) or unwanted pregnancy and previous sexual abuse.

Young women — deep dyspareunia
1 Infection — chlamydia infection with PID.
2 Endometriosis — deposits in uterosacral ligaments or rectovaginal septum.

Dyspareunia

3 No cause — often extensive investigation fails to elucidate a cause. Many of these are young women with family or relationship problems. Emotionally labile during consultation. May have had sexual abuse in the past. A '*crie de coeur*' for unresolved past conflicts.

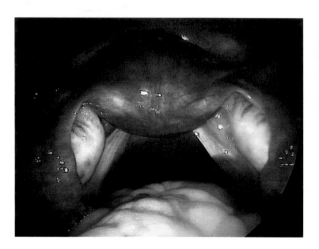

Fig 5.15 Twenty-six-year-old with dyspareunia. A negative laparoscopy. Admitted relationship problems with boyfriend who will not marry her.

Older women — superficial dyspareunia
1 Vaginal dryness — with narrow, shortened vagina.
2 Lichen sclerosis — atrophy and contracture of introitus.
3 Vaginismus — fear of penetration.
4 Vulvodynia — intense vaginal burning.

Older women — deep dyspareunia
1 Pelvic pathology — fibroids, cysts, pelvic malignancy.
2 Psychosexual problems — low libido, fear of penetration, guilt at 'letting partner down',

Dyspareunia

husband often 'too sympathetic', gynaecological surgery used as an excuse to terminate sexual responsibility.

Management
1 Treatment of infection.
2 Excision of scar tissue and vaginal introital reconstruction—Fenton's repair.
3 Exclusion of pathology by laparoscopy.
4 Attention to lubrication.
5 Oestrogen replacement therapy.
6 Psychosexual counselling. Some women just do not want to have sexual relationships and this needs to be recognised and accepted.

6 Fertility—infertility and contraception

Infertility

A common cause for consultations with both the GP and specialist affecting one in six couples.

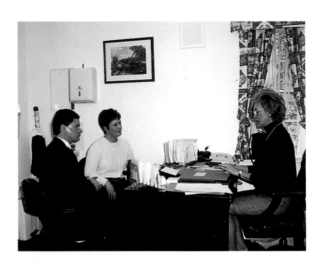

Fig 6.1 Couples with infertility need to be given realistic expectations of treatment and outcome.

Incidence

1 One in six couples will experience fertility problems.

2 80–90% of fertile couples will achieve a pregnancy within 12 months of trying and 95% within 2 years.

Aetiology

This is usually multifactorial and varies with the duration of infertility. At an early stage, it includes the following.

1 Unexplained infertility, 30% (really delayed normal fertility).

2 Male factor, 25% (single most common defined cause).

3 Ovulatory failure, 20%.

Infertility

4 Tubal damage, 15%
5 Endometriosis, 5%.

Management
1 Investigations can be completed in 2–3 months and the majority can be undertaken by the GP.
2 Referral to a specialist clinic can occur early for older, anxious women.
3 Younger women, in the absence of specific indications, can wait up to 2 years before referral for laparoscopy.

Special points

The GP holds the past records, has the patient's confidence, has a more flexible appointment system and can examine the male partner more easily than can the gynaecologist in the hospital clinic setting.

First visit

There is a lot to achieve in the first visit and time needs to be taken to ensure adequate assessment of the couple. The woman should attend with her partner, if possible, at this visit.
1 Take the couple's history with special reference to:
    (a) age and duration of infertility;
    (b) prior success of female partner;
    (c) past genital infections or surgery in either partner or intrauterine contraceptive device (IUD) usage;
    (d) medical conditions, such as diabetes, acne, hirsutism and galactorrhoea;
    (e) weight, smoking or alcohol problems;

Infertility

(f) pelvic pain and dyspareunia — *in which case refer early for laparoscopy*;

(g) impotence and coital frequency.

2 Pelvic examination, which should include:

(a) a cervical smear, if indicated;

(b) identification of an underlying pathological problem (e.g. fibroids or pelvic inflammatory disease (PID)) and tenderness.

3 Start a menstrual calendar.

4 Arrange a pelvic scan to check ovaries and follicle content.

5 Arrange follicle-stimulating hormone (FSH) and luteinising hormone (LH) assays on Day 5 of the cycle, and a rubella antibody titre. If menstrual irregularity exists, measure the serum level of thyroid-stimulating hormone (TSH) and prolactin level.

6 A mid luteal serum progesterone assay should be arranged on three cycles to check ovulatory status.

7 Advise on weight reduction if necessary, and recommend folic acid, 4 mg daily, to reduce neural tube abnormalities.

Special points

1 If the history and examination suggest recent or past pelvic chlamydial infection, an endocervical swab should be sent to the laboratory for a chlamydial immuno-fluorescence test.

2 If positive, both partners should be treated with ofloxacin.

Table 6.1 The World Health Organization's normal values for semen.

Parameter measured	Normal value
Semen volume	>2 ml
Sperm concentration	>20 million/ml
Sperm motility	50% with forward progression or more than 25% with rapid progression
Sperm	>30% with normal morphology

Infertility

8 A semen analysis (Table 6.1) should be arranged — 3 days' abstinence before collection with delivery to the laboratory within 2 hours. Repeat in 1 month.
9 Advise on the identification of the fertile period using mucus recognition or ovulation detection kits, e.g. Clear View®, First Response®.

Second visit

This should take place after 3 months to assess the results of the preliminary investigations.

Semen analysis
1 If this shows a reduction in count or motility on two samples taken 1 month apart, consider referral to andrologist or urologist.
2 The treatment of choice for men with sub-optimal sperm profiles is intracytoplasmic

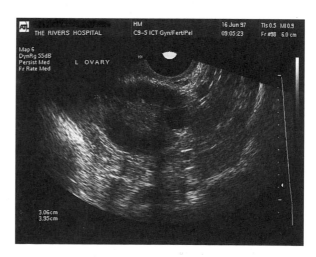

Fig 6.2 A pelvic scan will detect polycystic ovaries.

Infertility

sperm injection (ICSI). A single sperm is captured and injected into the cytoplasm of the oocyte to effect fertilisation. The technique is really only available in the private sector and the initial results are promising.

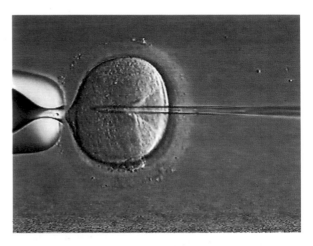

Fig 6.3 Micropipette inserting sperm into cytoplasm of ovum.

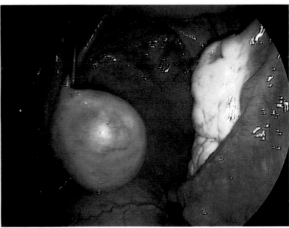

Fig 6.4 Preovulatory follicle on left ovary at Day 14.

Ovulatory status

1 If ovulation is occurring with progesterone

Infertility

levels of more than 30 nmol/l on three cycles, the woman can be reassured and, if older or anxious, can be referred to a specialist clinic for tubal assessment via the laparoscope.

2 Women with normal cycles are not treated with clomiphene citrate unless they have 3 years of unexplained infertility. Normal cycling women can be referred for laparoscopic assessment of the pelvis after 12–18 months.

3 Anovulation usually exists with low serum progesterone levels and irregular cycles. An attempt to induce ovulation can be made with clomiphene citrate, 50 mg daily, from Day 2 to Day 6 of the cycle for three cycles. Further progesterone level assays can be performed to monitor response. The dose of clomiphene citrate can be increased to 100 mg daily if the patient is unresponsive. This type of regimen is quite safe and appropriate for the GP to instigate and supervise.

Special points

1 If serum progesterone levels are low, check that they were measured within 10 days of the following period.
2 Cycle confusion can lead to inaccurate results.

Special notes on the use of clomiphene citrate

1 Menopausal symptoms may arise on clomiphene citrate therapy.
2 Oligomenorrhoeic women may need to induce a bleed with medroxyprogesterone acetate, 10 mg daily for 7 days, before starting clomiphene citrate treatment.
3 80% of women with polycystic ovaries will ovulate on clomiphene citrate: 30–50% will conceive.
4 Clomiphene citrate therapy is associated with a fivefold increase in the likelihood of having twins.
5 Miscarriage occurs in 20% of naturally conceived pregnancies. It is even more frequent in clomiphene citrate-stimulated cycles.

Infertility

Specialist clinic

If the couple fails to conceive after three to six cycles of clomiphene therapy, refer to specialist clinic which may carry out the following.

1 Make adjustments to drug therapy.
2 Perform a postcoital test.
3 Perform an ultrasound follicle-tracking scan.
4 Use laparoscopy to confirm tubal patency and normal ovaries and exclude adhesions and endometriosis.

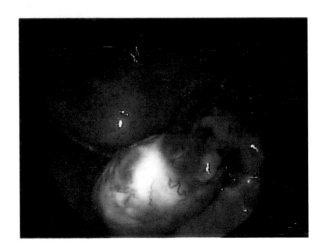

Fig 6.5 Patent tube on dye test.

5 Use definitive surgery via the laparoscope to treat endometriosis or induce ovulation in resistant cases of polycystic ovaries by multidiathermy.

Infertility

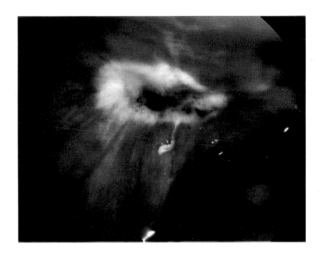

Fig 6.6 Diathermy to clear endometriosis.

6 Patients with pelvic pain, menorrhagia and dyspareunia should be referred early for specialist help to exclude endometriosis and tubal damage from chlamydial infection.

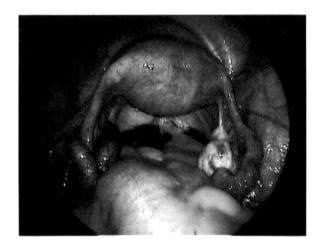

Fig 6.7 Pelvic damage — blocked side tube.

Infertility

7 Women with:

(a) an abnormal thyroid function test will need further assessment and treatment in an endocrine clinic;

(b) an abnormally raised prolactin level will need further investigation (see Chapter 2 for hyperprolactinaemia);

(c) a raised LH level (Day 5 of cycle, >10 IU/l) will require a transvaginal ultrasound scan to diagnose polycystic ovarian disease (see Chapter 2). The syndrome comprises oligomenorrhoea and/or obesity and hirsutism. Ovulation induction with clomiphene citrate is used and can be managed by the GP.

8 Following investigations, a large proportion of couples will be told that there is no obvious cause of their infertility and labelled as having 'unexplained infertility'. They may conceive naturally in the next 2 years, but this is a frustrating time; if they are not successful, *in vitro* fertilisation (IVF) and/or gamete intrafallopian transfer (GIFT) can be advised.

Assisted conception clinics

Techniques

Patients who have failed to conceive after 2 years of treatment, those with irreparable tubal damage and those who, for reasons of advancing age, request assisted conception can have the following treatments (see Table 6.2 for a comparison of the success rates of the techniques).

Gamete intrafallopian transfer (GIFT)
For prolonged unexplained infertility or endometriosis. Oocytes are harvested using

Infertility

Table 6.2 Assisted reproduction techniques.

	Approximate cost (£)*	Success rate	
		Pregnancy rate (%)	Live birth rate (%)
In vitro fertilisation (IVF)	2000	25	20
Gamete intrafallopian transfer (GIFT)	2000	35	30
Superovulation with intrauterine insemination (IUI)	500	15	12
Intracytoplasmic sperm injection (ICSI)	2500	25	20
Additional costs			
Stimulation drugs	500		
Cryopreservation requested	300		

*Costs may vary between clinics.

ultrasound and replaced into tube with pre-pared sperm by laparoscopy. Patent healthy tubes are necessary.

In vitro fertilisation (IVF)
For women with damaged fallopian tubes, endometriosis, prolonged unexplained infertility or if the sperm count is poor. The ovaries are stimulated to produce multiple eggs (oocytes), which are usually harvested by ultrasound-guided vaginal collection and fertilised in the laboratory with sperm; up to three are replaced in the uterine cavity. Spare embryos can be frozen for subsequent use.

Intracytoplasmic sperm injection (ICSI)
Couples in whom the male partner has a relatively severe sperm deficit or dysfunction can be

Infertility

treated with ICSI. This is a microtechnique which involves the insertion of a single sperm directly into the ovum's cytoplasm to achieve fertilisation and the replacement of the embryo into the uterus.

Intrauterine insemination (IUI)
Insemination with specially prepared husband or donor sperm into the uterus to overcome cervical problems or unexplained infertility. Usually combined with ovarian stimulation to induce multiple ovulation.

Contraception

Combined oral contraceptive pill (COCP)

25% of women in their reproductive years use this method and make frequent visits to their GP and family planning clinics for supplies.

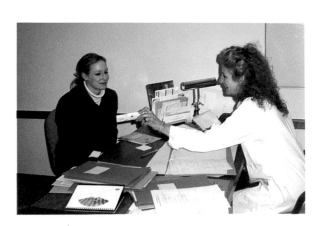

Fig 6.8 A popular method of contraception with many women.

Contraception

Advantages of the COCP

1 Menstrual periods are regular, lighter, less painful and premenstrual tension (PMT) may improve.

2 Acne and hirsutism—Dianette® recommended, but not licensed for contraception, although effective with good cycle control

3 Reduction in benign breast disorders.

4 Reduction in PID.

5 Reduction in ovarian cyst incidence.

6 Reduction in fibroid incidence.

7 Reduction in cancer of the ovary and endometrium.

8 Reduction in bacterial vaginosis and toxic shock syndrome.

9 Reduction in the incidence of thyroid disease, anaemia and duodenal ulcers.

Contraindications to the COCP

1 A personal history of venous thrombosis.

2 Gross obesity.

3 Immobility.

4 Breast cancer.

5 Heavy smoking and especially in women over 35 years of age.

6 A family history of venous thrombosis in women under 45 years of age, in siblings or parents. Investigate with Activated Protein C Resistance Test as a screen before starting the COCP.

7 Varicose veins—women with mild varicose veins may take the COCP.

8 The risk of venous thromboembolism and mortality in women as a result of oral contraceptive use is shown in Table 6.3.

Special points

Non-smokers over 40 years of age may now safely take the COCP up to the menopause. Low-dose oestrogen choice.

Contraception

Table 6.3 Risk of venous thromboembolism and mortality in women as a result of oral contraceptive use and pregnancy.*

	VTE per 100 000 women per year	Mortality per 1 million women per year
No OC use	5	0.5
Second-generation combined OC	15	1.5
Combined OC containing desogestrel and gestodene†	30	3
Pregnancy	60	6

OC, oral contraceptive; VTE, venous thromboembolism.

*Source: Medicines Control Agency, from various studies. Health Trends 1996; **28** (3).

†Following the report from the Committee on Safety of Medicine (CSM) in 1995, oral contraceptives containing gestodene and desogestrel were identified with an increased risk of venous thrombosis and mortality compared with second-generation pills. The absolute risk is very small and much smaller than the risk of pregnancy.

Special points

1 Women with a personal or family history of thrombosis may be screened for mutation of factor V Leiden before commencing the COCP. Presence of the mutation excludes COCP usage.

2 Third-generation pills—desogestrel and gestodene—provide protection against myocardial infarction and may be the best choice for smokers, diabetics and older, hypertensive women. They are also used for women who have side effects on second-generation pills.

Recommendations

Use the lowest oestrogen dose and a second-generation progestogen as first-line treatment.

1 Loestrin 20®, Parke-Davis.
2 Loestrin 30®, Parke-Davis.
3 Microgynon 30®, Schering HC.
4 Cilest®, Janssen-Cilag.
5 Ovranette®, Wyeth.

Contraception

Problems on the COCP

1 Weight gain—can have a gain of 5 lb (2.5 kg) in a few months, but usually lost again over ensuing months.

2 Headaches—contraindicated in women with focal migraine, crescendo migraine, first attack of migraine on the COCP and severe migraines requiring use of ergotamine.

3 Breakthrough bleeding—try a different progestogen or a triphasic pill and, if persists, refer to exclude pathology.

4 Forgotten pills:

(a) mid-cycle—low risk of pregnancy, can miss 4 days (ovary quiescent);

(b) end of pack—start next pack straight away without allowing seven pill-free days;

(c) start of pack—*danger period*—after seven pill-free days, further omission may allow escape ovulation. Advise to continue pill taking—use a condom for that cycle or for 7 days after last missed pill.

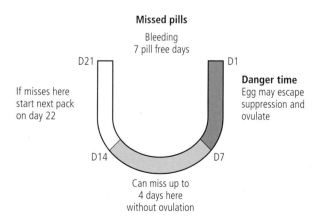

Fig 6.9 Missed pills.

Contraception

5 Surgery—discontinue for 4 weeks prior to major surgery or leg surgery. Progestogen-only pill can be substituted. Recommence after full mobilisation during subsequent normal period.
6 Emergency surgery—discontinue and cover operation with heparin prophylaxis.

Special points

There is no association between vaginal candidiasis and the use of low- to medium-dose oestrogen oral contraceptives.

Progestogen-only pill

This type of pill is used by 5% of women taking pill contraception and is also called the 'mini pill'. It thickens the cervical mucus to prevent sperm penetration and causes anovulatory cycles in 60% of patients.
1 It *must* be taken at the same time each day, usually early evenings, and taken *continuously*.
2 If forgotten for more than 3 h, a barrier method should be used for 7 days.
3 If unprotected sexual intercourse occurs after 3 h, emergency contraception must be considered.

Products available
1 Micronor® or Noriday®, which contain 0.35 mg norethisterone.
2 Femulen®, which contains 0.5 mg ethynodiol diacetate.
3 Microval® or Norgeston®, which contain 0.075 mg norgestrel.

Contraception

Indications
1 Breast-feeding mothers.
2 Diabetic women.
3 Severe focal migraine sufferers.
4 Women with increased risk of thromboembolism due to:
    (a) inherited disorders;
    (b) immobility;
    (c) major surgery.
5 Women with increased risk of cardiovascular disease, for example:
    (a) smokers over 35 years of age;
    (b) hypertensives;
    (c) women with hyperlipidaemia.
6 Women who experience symptoms on the COCP from the oestrogen component.
7 At woman's request.

Contraindications
Women with a previous history of the following.
1 Ectopic pregnancy.
2 Ovarian cysts.
Otherwise the progestogen-only pill is very safe.

Management required
When starting the progestogen-only pill, it is important, especially if the woman is under 25 years of age (due to their higher failure rate), to undertake the following.
1 Give the patient precise verbal instructions.
2 Give written instructions to support conversation.
3 Offer further appointments in 3 months to reassess, and warn of breakthrough bleeding which occurs but settles with duration of use.

Special points
1 Younger obese women over 70 kg should take two tablets daily.
2 Poor cycle control is a problem and so not suitable for adolescents.

Contraception

If problems are present, try a different progestogen.

Injectable contraceptives

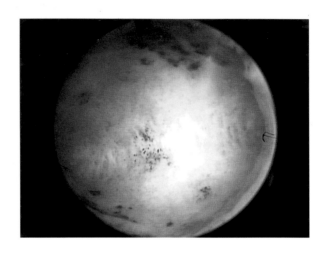

Fig 6.10 Atrophic endometrium in a 17-year-old school girl on Depo-Provera®.

Depo-Provera®
1 Contains 17α-hydroxyprogesterone (150 mg/ml).
2 Given by deep intramuscular injection into deltoid or gluteus muscle.
3 Inexpensive.
4 Needs to be repeated every 12 weeks.
5 The first injection is given during the first 5 days of menstruation.
6 Safe and effective.

Advantages
1 Can be used for breast-feeding women.
2 Useful for patients with poor compliance on other methods.
3 No interaction with antibiotics.
4 Reduces dysmenorrhoea and menorrhagia and the incidence of ovarian cysts.

Contraception

5 Reduces the incidence of PID.
6 Controls premenstrual aggression in educationally subnormal women and relieves PMT.
7 Failure rate of only 1% per 100 women years.
8 Useful for women with sickle-cell disease.

Disadvantages
1 Once injected cannot be removed.
2 Weight gain and acne can occur.
3 Prolonged breakthrough bleeding can be a problem.
4 Amenorrhoea—55% will have no periods by the end of the first year—may be an advantage!
5 Delay in return of fertility for approximately 6 months, but no permanent effect.

Special points

Modern career women appreciate the absence of periods and relief from PMT that all the Depo progestogens provide.

Noristerat®
1 Given as a 200 mg/ml deep intramuscular injection into the gluteus muscle.
2 First injection is given during menstruation.
3 Needs to be repeated every 8 weeks, but better cycle control than Depo-Provera®.
4 Useful for short-term, highly efficacious contraception in, for example:
   (a) postpartum women awaiting sterilisation;

Contraception

(b) partners of men awaiting vasectomy;
(c) after rubella immunisation.

Contraceptive implants

Norplant®
1 Consists of six Silastic rods containing levo-norgestrel which are inserted subdermally under local anaesthetic and last 5 years.
2 Requires trained personnel to insert and remove device.
3 This method is no longer popular and few GPs offer the method owing to unwanted side effects.
4 Implanon a new single rod desogestrel releasing implant will soon be available.

Intrauterine contraceptive devices (IUDs)

Recommended products
The third-generation, copper-releasing devices.
1 Ortho Gyne-T® 380 Slimline.
2 Multiload® Cu375.
For specific details of the products, see Table 6.4.

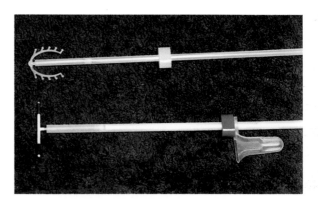

Fig 6.11 IUDs: Multiload® Cu375 and Ortho Gyne-T® 380 Slimline.

Contraception

Table 6.4 Details of the recommended IUDs. These are compared with the intrauterine system Mirena®.

Product	Approximate failure rate (% women years)	Recommended retrieval interval (years)	Cost (£)	Cost per month of use (£)
Multiload® Cu375	0.9	5+	9.62	0.16
Ortho Gyne-T® 380 Slimline	0.4	8+	9.40	0.10
Mirena®*	0.2	3+	99.65	2.76

*See intrauterine system (IUS) (see next section).
The GyneFIX® intrauterine implant system is now available. Frameless and flexible, it is fixed to the fundus of the uterus. Good tolerance and non-expulsion are reported.

Advantages
1 Highly effective. The pregnancy rate is vary low—0.3 per 100 women years.
2 A cheap 'fit and forget' contraceptive. Costs £10.00. Low expulsion rate as 'fundal seeking'.
3 Efficacy lasts 8 years.
4 Women over 40 years of age being fitted can retain the device *in situ* until 1 year after the menopause without changing.
5 Easy to insert—usually during menstruation.
6 Can be used for emergency contraception for up to 5 days after possible ovulation—Day 19 of cycle.
7 Low rates of ectopic pregnancy with these devices.

Disadvantages
1 Pain—insertion may be uncomfortable and warrant a local anaesthetic cervical block.

Contraception

2 Periods—moderate increase in monthly blood of about 30 ml at 12 months, but no change in iron status observed. Occasional intermenstrual and postcoital bleeding.

3 Lost threads—most can be retrieved from the canal with a plastic thread retriever or curved Spencer Wells forceps. Only 4% of women will require anaesthetic to remove IUD. Scan to check location in intrauterine cavity is advised.

4 PID—extensive trials have shown a low risk of this following insertion of the IUD: 0.2%.

5 Special points to note are as follows.

(a) The IUD needs a sterile method of insertion.

(b) It should be used in women who show no signs of infection, because during insertion organisms may ascend the genital tract. Chlamydial infection is present in 6–8% of women attending family planning clinics and, as it can be symptomless, may require a special screening test to determine whether it is present.

(c) At risk groups include young, sexually active women and those with multiple sexual partners.

(d) Antibiotic cover should be considered if any suspicion of chlamydial infection or if fitted for emergency contraception, and early review within 6 weeks of fitting should be undertaken to allow any PID to be diagnosed and managed promptly. The greatest incidence occurs within 20 days of device insertion.

Contraception

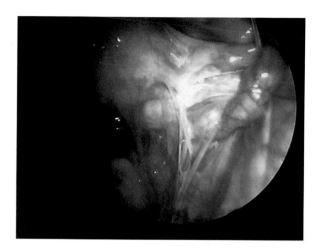

Fig 6.12 Silent chlamydial infection after IUD insertion.

6 If *Actinomyces* is found on routine smear and
(a) the patient is asymptomatic, remove IUD and reinsert after 3 months if smear is normal; no antibiotics needed;
(b) the patient is symptomatic (pelvic tenderness), remove IUD and send for culture, swab endocervix and refer the patient to genitourinary medicine (GUM) clinic for treatment with high-dosage penicillin.
A cervical smear is recommended 6 months after IUD insertion and yearly thereafter to check for *Actinomyces*-like organisms.

7 Pregnancy. If the woman conceives with an IUD, gently remove the device at the earliest opportunity. Early removal decreases the incidence of pregnancy loss and complications from 54% to 20%. Ectopic pregnancy should be excluded.

8 Perforation. This is rare (1 : 1000 insertions) and is usually painless. The threads disappear

Contraception

and an ultrasound scan will be required to confirm the location of the IUD. Will need laparoscopy or laparotomy for retrieval.

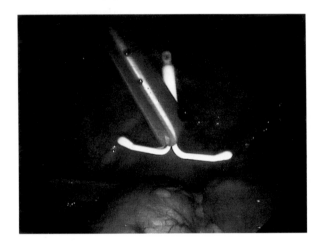

Fig 6.13 IUD can perforate the uterus and need retrieval via the laparoscope.

Management
1 The IUD should be fitted by experienced, trained doctors.
2 Patients should be followed up 6 weeks later to ensure that threads are visible and there is no pelvic infection.
3 Six-monthly check is recommended thereafter.

Intrauterine system (IUS)

The levonorgestrel IUS (Mirena® IUS), which is marketed as Mirena®, was launched in May 1995.
1 It releases 20 µg levonorgestrel daily.
2 It is extremely safe and efficient. The pregnancy rate is 0.2 per 100 women years.

Contraception

3 It has a low ectopic pregnancy rate and can be used in women with previous ectopic pregnancy.
4 It has a 3-year duration of action, but a licence for 5 years is applied for.
5 Menses are lighter and less painful.
6 It is associated with a reduced risk of pelvic infection.
7 It is 100% reversible—conception rate 79–96% within 12 months.

Disadvantages
1 It requires a thicker insertion tube than other IUDs (4.5 mm) and may need local anaesthetic and dilation in nulliparous women.
2 Irregular bleeding for 3 months, but amenorrhoea in 10% of women after 12 months. Mild progestogenic symptoms can occur.
3 Costs £100.00.

Special notes

1 An 'ideal contraceptive', but women need counselling about initial erratic bleeding and spotting.
2 Oestrogen levels in women with amenorrhoea are not low.

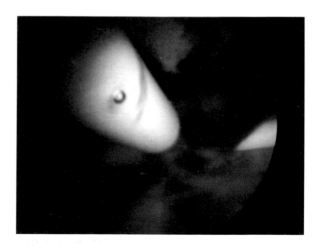

Fig 6.14 The Mirena® IUS in the uterine cavity.

Contraception

Indications
1 Women with menorrhagia.
2 Women with mental or physical handicap.
3 Older women who smoke and are diabetic or hypertensive.
4 Women in whom combined oral contraceptives are contraindicated.
5 Women requesting termination of pregnancy where other methods of contraception have failed.

Female sterilisation

Increasingly popular method of contraception; 45% of couples in their forties have been sterilised—either male or female. The object of this operation is to occlude the fallopian tubes permanently in order to prevent sperm reaching and fertilising the ovum. It is a popular, very effective method for women over 30 years of age who have completed their families. It should be regarded as irreversible.

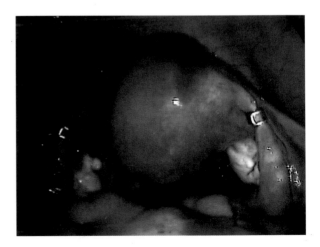

Fig 6.15 The Filshie clip applied to and occluding the fallopian tubes.

Contraception

Advantages
1 Permanent 'one-off' method.
2 Menstrual function is not changed despite the belief that periods become heavier.
3 A day-case procedure, although it usually requires a general anaesthetic, but can be performed under a local anaesthetic.

Disadvantages
1 Failure rate of 4 per 1000.
2 If failure occurs, there may be an ectopic rate of 5%.

Recommendations
1 Couples should be counselled on the advantages of vasectomy, i.e. it is safer, cheaper and just as effective. Many men are resistant to the idea.
2 Filshie clips are used as there are fewer perioperative complications and the procedure is more likely to be reversible.
3 Couples should be counselled on the failure rate, ectopic rate and intended permanency, with good documentation.
4 The procedure should not be performed on recently pregnant women in association with abortion as the incidence of regret is increased and the failure rate is much higher.

Contraception

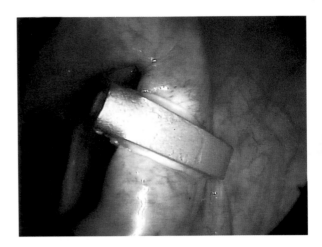

Fig 6.16 Reversal of sterilisation may be possible as tubal destruction is minimal.

Special notes

1 In the event of a reversal request, the success of tubal reanastomosis and subsequent conception is about 80%, provided that Filshie clips have been used and placed in the middle of the tube.

2 The old-fashioned Pomeroy procedure removed much of the fallopian tube during open surgery, and these women have a low success rate for reanastomosis as it is difficult to reconstruct a functional length.

3 Failure of laparoscopic sterilisation remains one of the major causes of medicolegal litigation, and detailed counselling is required before the procedure is undertaken.

Barrier methods of contraception

The existence of the human immunodeficiency virus (HIV) has increased the popularity of barrier methods. The 'Double Dutch' method is safest and should be widely practised—it involves the use of both oral contraception to inhibit ovulation and a condom to prevent sexu-

Contraception

ally transmitted diseases (STDs). 70% of people choose to obtain their contraception from GPs and free condoms should be available. All couples should be encouraged to use this method.

Male condom
18% of couples use this method.
1 Made from latex, and therefore can deteriorate and split if used with vaseline or baby oil as a lubricant.
2 Widely used and very popular.
3 Young men may need demonstration of application.
4 A slimline condom is available and Durex Avanti, a polyurethane, is now available.

Female condom
1 Made from polyurethane and so not damaged by lubricants.
2 Good protection against STDs.
3 Crackles during sexual intercourse.

Diaphragms and caps
Reducing in popularity because of the following.
1 Messy and need a spermicidal cream as well.
2 Require premeditation.
3 Can cause bladder irritability.
4 Have a high failure rate: 12 per 100 women years.
5 Removing a cap may be even more difficult than insertion because the suction seal has to be broken.

Special points

Condoms provide excellent protection against many sexually transmitted infections.

Contraception

6 Require special size fitting by trained personnel.
However, some women like the method and the control it gives them.

Natural methods of contraception

Temperature charts, cervical mucus and ovulation pain have been used in the past by women to detect their fertile period and restrict sexual intercourse at that time. Persona®, a monoclonal antibody test to detect imminent ovulation, has become popular 'over the counter'.

Contraception and the older woman

Reduced fertility after 35 years of age. Smokers must stop combined oral contraception at 35 years of age. Healthy, non-smoking women of 40 years of age and over can choose from the following.

1 COCP—stop at 50 years of age and use a barrier method to determine menopausal status (flushing, etc.):
    (a) Loestrin 20®;
    (b) Cilest®;
    (c) Mercilon®.

2 Progestogen-only pill:
    (a) Micronor®;
    (b) Femulen®.

3 IUD: Ortho Gyne-T® 380 Slimline, which should remain in place until 1 year postmenopause.

4 IUS: levonorgestrel IUS (Mirena®). Effective for 5 years, but can probably leave *in situ* until after the menopause. Most will become amen-

Contraception

orrhoeic when using this method. The woman should be warned of spotting during the first 3 months.

5 Laparoscopic sterilisation: many request this as a definitive method after 'near accidents'.

Emergency contraception

Oral medication

For use within 72 h of unprotected sexual intercourse.

1 Ovran 50® — four tablets immediately and, if vomiting occurs within 3 h, give another two tablets.

2 Schering PC4® — two tablets and repeat in 12 h; if vomiting occurs within 3 h, give a further two tablets. Failure rate: 2–8%.

3 Levonorgestrel — 0.75 mg stat., and repeat in 12 h for women in whom oestrogen is a contraindication or who have rejected an IUD. Use on named patient basis and within 72 h of unprotected sexual intercourse. Examples are:

    (a) Microval® — 25 tablets stat., and repeat in 12 h;

    (b) Neogest® — 20 tablets stat., and repeat in 12 h.

Contraindications:

1 current focal migraine;

2 proven venous thrombosis;

3 porphyria;

4 jaundice.

Contraception

IUD insertion

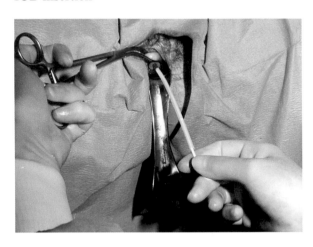

Fig 6.17 Insertion of an IUD.

Special points

Recommended IUDs:
Ortho Gyne-T® 380
Slimline, Janssen-Cilag;
Multiload® Cu250 Short,
Organon.

1 Prevents three out of four pregnancies, and the device can be inserted up to 5 days after the calculated ovulation date on the individual's cycle length, despite the number of episodes of unprotected sexual intercourse.

2 Can be left in place for ongoing contraception or removed after next period ensues.

3 If the pregnancy is ongoing, termination should not be recommended on the grounds of fetal abnormality. The risk is very low.

4 The woman needs a follow-up appointment to check her pregnancy status and to discuss effective contraception for the future. Many are young girls who have had their first sexual experience, and others are older women with contraceptive failure who might be suitable for definitive sterilisation.

Contraception

Postnatal contraception

Breast-feeding mothers
1 Progestogen-only pill, start at 4 weeks.
2 Injectables, start at 4 weeks.
3 IUD, fit at 6 weeks.
4 Mirena® IUS, fit at 6 weeks.

Special points

If the woman has had a caesarean section, fit the IUD at 3 months' postpartum.

Non-breast-feeding mothers
1 COCP, start at 3 weeks.
2 Progestogen-only pill, start at 3 weeks.
3 Injectables, start at 3 weeks.
4 IUD, fit at 6 weeks.
5 Mirena® IUS, fit at 6 weeks.

Contraception for the teenager

Girls in their mid-teens need frank and open counselling about contraception. One in ten 15-year-old girls are reported to be taking the contraceptive pill in the UK.

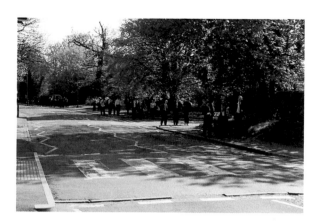

Fig 6.18 Teenagers have special need for advice and help.

153

Contraception

1 They have extensive information on sexual intercourse from magazines which focus on this age group, from explicit television programmes and from education in schools.

2 Sexual taboos and the preservation of virginity have ceased to be important in Western society. Many parents openly condone sexual activity in school children. Peer group pressure is intense.

3 Many young people have money to fund a social life that involves alcohol, soft drugs and 'clubbing'. Alcohol is probably responsible for the lessening of sexual inhibitions.

4 Many young girls have unprotected sexual intercourse and then seek advice on contraception, and many do not want their mothers to know about contraceptive pill taking.

5 A request for emergency contraception is an ideal opportunity to discuss and plan future contraception.

6 Many young women present with a request for contraception when they fear that they have contracted a genital infection. They need examination and reassurance. The fear of STD is widespread, and the opportunity to provide information about protection should not be missed.

7 Advise the young and all women entering into new sexual relationships to use both condoms and hormonal contraception.

8 Advise on emergency contraception. Information on what to do if pills are missed must accompany explicit instructions on:
    (a) when to start the contraceptive pill;
    (b) how to take them correctly;

Contraception

(c) the best time to take them to prevent forgotten pills.

Methods suitable for the young girl

A very positive approach to the advantages of the contraceptive pill can be adopted, and reassurance can be given that weight gain is transitory.

1 Oral contraceptive pill if she feels she can remember to take it each day.

(a) Microgynon® or Cilest®.

(b) Dianette® is very popular as it is good for acne which is a big problem at this age; this often ensures compliance.

Special notes

Antibiotics affect contraceptive pill absorption and the teenager should be warned to use additional protection if antibiotics are prescribed. Teenagers on long-term antibiotics are safe after 1 month of therapy.

---

2 Injectable contraception. Depo-Provera® can be offered with confidence. May become amenorrhoeic, which is welcomed, but advice should be given on slight, bloodstained discharge which can occur. Three-monthly injections are convenient and the method is reliable. Secrecy is afforded by this method.

Special notes

The IUD is unsuitable as many teenage girls have heavy, painful periods, risk STD from serial monogamy and being so fertile have a higher failure rate.

7 Fibroids—uterine leiomyoma

Fibroids—uterine leiomyoma, 158

Fibroids—uterine leiomyoma

The commonest pathological growth found in the uterus is a *fibroid*.

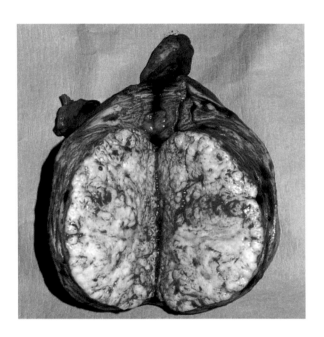

Fig 7.1 Discrete fibrous lumps called leiomyomas that arise in the myometrium and can grow under hormonal stimulation to a large size.

Incidence
About 20% of women will have small fibroids often detected incidentally on ultrasound. They may be multiple or solitary and vary in size.

Aetiology
Unknown, but commoner in low-parity women and there is some familial incidence.

Symptoms
1 Often none.
2 Menorrhagia if submucous in site.
3 Dysmenorrhoea if intracavity in site.

Fibroids — uterine leiomyoma

4 May contribute to infertility.

5 May cause pressure on bladder or backache if large and depending on site.

6 May undergo red degeneration and cause severe pain.

7 May dilate and prolapse through the cervix if polypoid and located in lower segment of uterus.

8 May be felt on abdominal palpation.

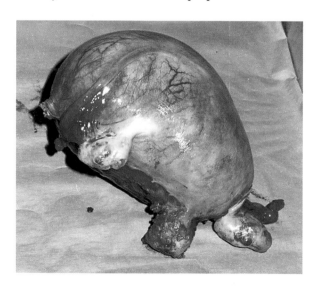

Fig 7.2 Hysterectomy performed on a patient presenting with urinary retention and impacted pelvic fibroid.

Management

1 Exclude pregnancy.

2 Check haemoglobin if menorrhagia is a symptom.

3 Pelvic ultrasound to confirm diagnosis and exclude ovarian mass.

4 Explanation of the benign nature.

5 Medical treatment.

    (a) Gonadotrophin-releasing agonists can be

Fibroids—uterine leiomyoma

used for short-term management to reduce the size prior to surgery.

(b) The oestrogen deficiency state that results from this treatment, e.g. vasomotor symptoms and vaginal dryness, is unacceptable to most women.

(c) Embolisation under radiological control is being tried. Results are awaited.

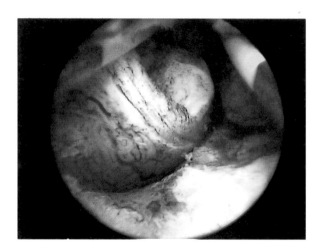

Fig 7.3 Hysteroscopic resection of intracavity fibroid.

6 Surgical treatment.

(a) Intracavity or submucous fibroids can be resected via the hysteroscope.

(b) Intramural or subserosal fibroids can be enucleated laparoscopically—cut up (morcellated) and removed via the laparoscope.

(c) Younger women may request a myomectomy to preserve the uterus for future childbearing; the procedure may be performed laparoscopically or at laparotomy depending

Fibroids—uterine leiomyoma

on the size, location, number of fibroids and surgical preference of the surgeon.

(d) Older women are advised to consider a total hysterectomy which can be performed abdominally or vaginally if size will permit.

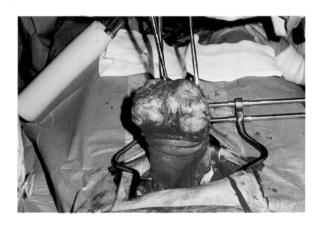

Fig 7.4 Myomectomy via open laparotomy in a nulliparous 30-year-old woman.

7 Treatment of fibroids by embolisation.

(a) Initial studies have begun on the treatment of fibroids by embolisation of the uterine artery to cause avascular necrosis and shrinkage of the fibroid.

(b) This option may appeal to women with symptomatic fibroids who do not wish to undergo surgical treatment by myomectomy or hysterectomy.

(c) Percutaneous femoral catheterisation is undertaken under sedation in the radiology department by radiologists experienced in angiography. The uterine artery is embolised to the occlusion of flow by injecting polyvinyl alcohol particles.

Fibroids—uterine leiomyoma

(d) Women needed admission for pain relief after the procedure, and variable results were obtained. Overall satisfaction was adequate. Intermittent pain, extrusion of avascular fibroids and ovarian failure were cited at follow-up.

(e) A larger series will be needed to assess patient selection, tolerance and results, as well as radiation exposure and subsequent fertility.

Special points

1 Hormone replacement therapy (HRT) is not contraindicated in postmenopausal women with fibroids.
2 Some women are content to live with large abdominal fibroids provided that they remain symptomless.
3 Women can be reassured that malignant change is very rare.

8 Ovarian cysts

Ovarian cysts — general, 164

Types of ovarian cyst, 167
Physiological or simple cysts, 167
Polycystic ovaries, 168
Endometriomas, 169
Germ cell tumours — dermoids, 171
Epithelial cysts — cystadenomas, 172
Solid ovarian growths, 173
Borderline tumours, 174

Ovarian cysts—general

These are common, frequently asymptomatic and often resolve spontaneously.

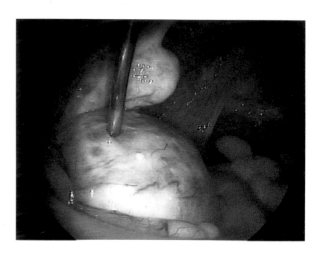

Fig 8.1 Large cyst on left ovary at laparoscopy.

Incidence

1 The ovary is a cystic structure and benign cystic change is normal in many healthy women.
2 Large or pathological cysts can occur in about 5% of women during their reproductive years, but many are not diagnosed unless they cause pain or abdominal distension.
3 Ovarian cysts are commonly diagnosed by ultrasonographers scanning young women for pelvic pain or menstrual irregularity. They will report follicular cysts or polycystic ovaries.

Aetiology

No consistent factor is accountable for the various diverse types of ovarian cyst.

Ovarian cysts — general

Symptoms

1 Often asymptomatic.

2 Mild menstrual irregularity and vague pelvic pain.

3 Low abdominal swelling.

4 Pain if torsion, rupture or haemorrhage occurs.

5 Amenorrhoea, obesity and hirsutism may be presenting symptoms.

6 Occasionally, dyspareunia may be the presenting symptom.

Special points

Women may be emotional about the diagnosis of an ovarian cyst and may need to discuss the impact of the diagnosis on future child-bearing and the likelihood of malignancy. The former is seldom affected and the latter is rare.

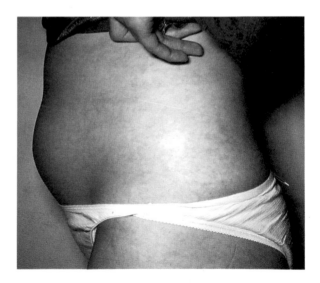

Fig 8.2 Rapid lower abdominal enlargement in a young woman suggests a cyst.

Ovarian cysts — general

Diagnosis

1 Exclude pregnancy and a full bladder.

2 Palpate the abdomen.

3 Perform a bimanual examination to detect cysts lying in the pouch of Douglas. Ovaries usually lie posterior to the uterus — cysts may be slippery and mobile and are often missed.

4 Pelvic ultrasound examination.

5 Severe pain usually indicates torsion or haemorrhage, and necessitates urgent referral to the casualty department for diagnosis and assessment by laparoscopy or laparotomy. Symptoms may mimic an ectopic pregnancy and this condition needs to be excluded.

6 Signs of virilisation should be sought, e.g. alopecia, hirsutism and clitoral hypertrophy, and, if present, would demand early referral for specialist investigation to exclude virilising ovarian tumours.

7 The diagnosis can lead to anxiety and time to discuss is helpful.

Special points

Occasionally women on clomiphene or gonadotrophin therapy for ovulation induction present with acute ovarian enlargement as part of the hyperstimulation syndrome.

Types of ovarian cyst

Physiological or simple cysts

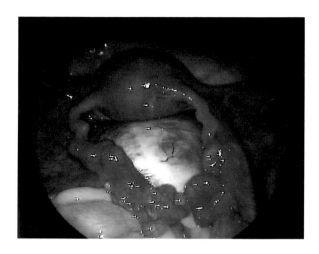

Fig 8.3 Physiological or simple cyst of right ovary filling pouch of Douglas.

Management

1 Follicular or corpus luteal cysts can develop, and may become quite large before resolving spontaneously.

2 Haemorrhage may occur into a corpus luteal cyst and present with delayed menstruation and sharp adnexal pain.

3 Ectopic pregnancy needs to be excluded.

4 Diagnosis, assessment and aspiration at laparoscopy are the correct management with follow-up ultrasonography to ensure resolution.

5 Cytology on the aspirate is reassuring and usually contains blood, macrophages, corpus luteum cells and/or follicular cells in a yellow fluid.

Special points

All women over the age of 35 years with ovarian enlargement and cystic change should be referred for further investigation and a blood test for the tumour marker Ca125.

Types of ovarian cyst

Polycystic ovaries

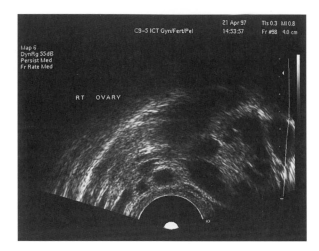

Fig 8.4 Ultrasound showing 'necklace' effect in ovary.

Special points

Medical management of the endocrine problems associated with the condition is required.

Management

1 Common and described in Chapter 2.

2 Enlarged bilateral ovaries with 'necklace' effect of small follicular cysts around the periphery and increased stroma on ultrasound.

3 At laparoscopy, large, pale, rubbery and inactive looking ovaries are seen.

4 Surgical intervention is rarely needed in this group. When fertility is an issue and persistent anovulation occurs, ovarian multidiathermy to induce ovulation is recommended.

Types of ovarian cyst

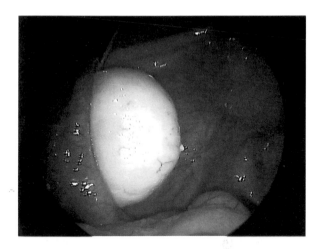

Fig 8.5 Laparoscopic view of large, pale, polycystic ovary.

Endometriomas

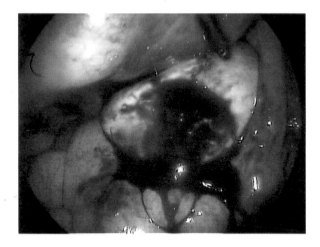

Fig 8.6 The chocolate cyst seen at laparoscopy.

Management

1 These blood-filled cysts arise in the ovary from the inclusion of endometrium into the ovarian structure.

2 Patients present with features of pelvic

Types of ovarian cyst

endometriosis, such as menorrhagia, infertility and pelvic pain. The diagnosis can be made by pelvic ultrasonography.

3 The ovaries are enlarged and there may be septa between smaller blood collections.

4 Careful laparoscopic appraisal and surgery are required to clear the tissues and conserve fertility.

5 Puncture of the cyst releases thick, chocolate-like fluid. The rest of the pelvis may show endometriotic deposits.

Special points

Ultrasonography may be helpful, but can be unreliable sometimes at diagnosing endometriomas and malignancy.

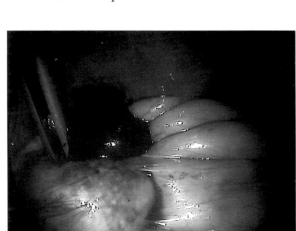

Fig 8.7 Endometrioma of left ovary — note adhesions to bowel.

Types of ovarian cyst

Germ cell tumours — dermoids

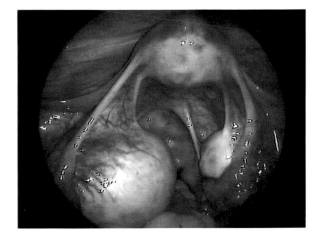

Fig 8.8 A view at laparoscopy of a dermoid cyst.

Management

1 The commonest type of pathological cyst in young women.

2 Usually symptomless; often diagnosed in early pregnancy.

3 Can be bilateral in 12% of cases, grow to 15 cm and contain a variety of tissue, mostly fat and hair, but teeth, bone, thyroid and cartilage can be present.

4 Low malignancy rate — 3%.

5 Should be removed by laparotomy or laparoscopy in skilled hands.

6 Prone to torsion.

Types of ovarian cyst

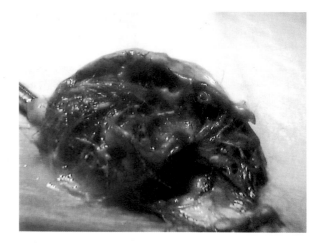

Fig 8.9 The cyst opened up — a large, hairy dermoid.

Epithelial cysts — cystadenomas

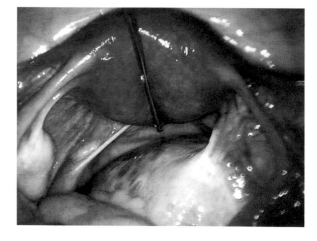

Fig 8.10 A large, epithelial cyst on right ovary.

Management

1 These cysts grow from epithelial ovarian structures and can become quite large.

2 They may contain many litres of fluid.

    (a) The *serous* variety is filled with pale yellow fluid and is the most common benign tumour.

Types of ovarian cyst

(b) The *mucinous* variety is filled with a gelatinous, slimy mucin—20% of all ovarian tumours.

3 Once diagnosed they need to be removed, usually by laparotomy or laparoscopy and excision of the cyst wall, otherwise they tend to recur. The ovary may be preserved by careful dissection.

4 Care must be taken to prevent the spill of mucin into the peritoneal cavity during removal as this may lead to pseudomyxoma peritonei.

5 These cysts in young women are seldom malignant, and therefore ovarian cystectomy or unilateral oophorectomy is appropriate to conserve fertility.

6 Women over 45 years of age with a cyst over 5 cm in diameter, or any other type of ovarian tumour, should be advised to undergo hysterectomy and bilateral oophorectomy.

Special points

1 These cysts may develop a pedicle and undergo torsion.
2 The woman then presents with severe pain and requires urgent investigation and treatment.

Solid ovarian growths

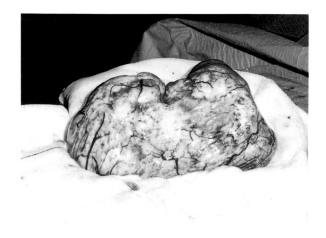

Fig 8.11 A 20-cm fibrothecoma of ovary in 44-year-old woman, exteriorised at laparotomy.

Types of ovarian cyst

Management

1 Much less common.

2 Often mistaken for a fibroid on clinical examination.

3 Can become very large with presure effects on the bladder.

4 After diagnosis, laparotomy is needed for removal and histological appraisal.

Borderline tumours

1 Women who have a diagnosis of a borderline tumour have an excellent prognosis regardless of the treatment given.

2 They are not precursors to ovarian cancer.

9 Genital prolapse or procidentia

Genital prolapse or procidentia, 176

Genital prolapse or procidentia

Cystourethrocele is the commonest type of prolapse, followed by uterine descent and rectocele.

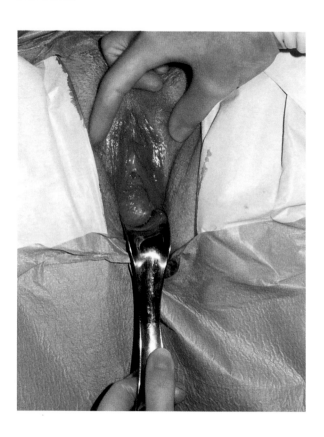

Fig 9.1 First-degree descent — cystourethrocele; 50% of patients with stress incontinence have this.

Incidence
About 20% of patients on waiting lists for gynaecological surgery are suffering from prolapse-related conditions.

Aetiology
1 Childbirth with pelvic floor damage from

Genital prolapse or procidentia

large babies, long labours and instrument deliveries.

2 Menopausal pelvic atrophy and collagen weakness.

3 Chronic cough or abdominal pressure and constipation.

Symptoms

1 Patient feels a lump coming down and may experience coital difficulty and backache.

2 Dragging pelvic sensation especially at the end of the day.

3 Concomitant stress incontinence or frequency, inadequate emptying and urinary tract infection (UTI).

4 Difficulty in defaecation and constipation.

5 Blood-stained discharge if prolapse rubs on underwear.

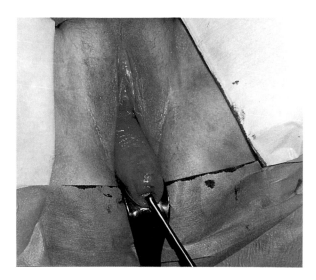

Fig 9.2 Second-degree descent of the cervix and uterus.

Genital prolapse or procidentia

Types of prolapse
1 Cystourethrocele — anterior vaginal wall prolapse.
2 Uterine descent — cervix may be seen in introital area.
3 Rectocele — posterior wall prolapse.
4 Combinations occur and, after a hysterectomy, the vagina may evert and hang out of the vulva — vault prolapse.
5 Enterocele — small bowel loops can herniate into the prolapsed areas.

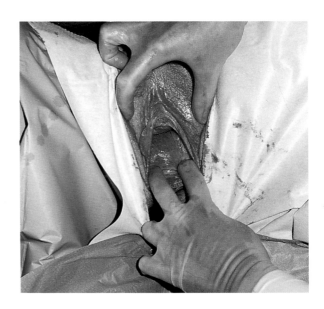

Fig 9.3 A rectocele prior to surgical repair.

Diagnosis
1 Diagnosed clinically. In the dorsal position with the thighs abducted and the labia parted, the patient is asked to cough or bear down. The

Genital prolapse or procidentia

prolapse can usually be seen. In the left lateral position and using a Sims speculum to retract the posterior wall, an anterior wall prolapse can be viewed.

2 A bimanual examination of the pelvis is performed to exclude a pelvic or abdominal mass, and a cervical smear may be indicated.

Management of prolapse

1 If patient is elderly, unfit or not keen on surgery, a *ring pessary* can be tried with local oestrogen cream or pessaries to prevent discharge and excoriation.

2 Start with small sizes and work up to obtain a good fit. Average is 71 mm.

3 Large prolapses in the elderly are better suited to support with a Simpson shelf pessary.

4 Pessaries only have to be changed yearly, but can give rise to vaginal discharge and excoriation of the vaginal epithelium.

5 Sexual intercourse with a pessary *in situ* may be uncomfortable.

6 In early pregnancy or for women desiring further pregnancies, ring pessaries are advised.

Genital prolapse or procidentia

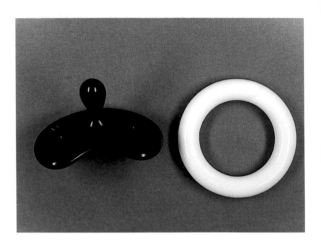

Fig 9.4 The Simpson shelf pessary and the ring pessary.

Surgery

Prior to surgery, oestrogen therapy will improve tissue quality.

1 Young women prefer a surgical repair, but may consent to a ring pessary whilst awaiting admission.

2 A cystocele can be corrected by an *anterior colporrhaphy — anterior repair.*

3 A rectocele can be corrected by a *posterior colpoperineorrhaphy — posterior repair.*

4 Uterine descent can be corrected by a *vaginal hysterectomy* and, if a cystocele or rectocele is also present, a *pelvic floor repair* will be performed.

5 Suprapubic catheters are used frequently to alleviate postoperative voiding problems.

6 If the vagina is hanging down after a previous hysterectomy (vault prolapse), a *sacro- colpopexy* is performed, whereby the vault is stitched to a mersilene graft that is suspended to

Genital prolapse or procidentia

the sacral promontory, pulling the vagina up inside.

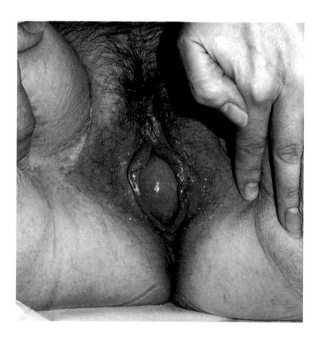

Fig 9.5 Vault prolapse after a hysterectomy.

7 Some of these procedures can be done laparoscopically, and transvaginal sacrospinous colpopexy is being assessed for vault prolapse.

Special points

1 If stress incontinence is present, a Burch colposuspension is preferred to an anterior repair.
2 After a posterior repair, there is an increased incidence of dyspareunia.

10 Urinary problems

Bacterial cystitis

A common infection in women, accounting for 6% of GP consultations.

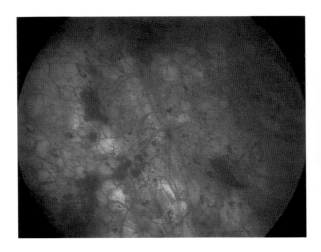

Fig 10.1 Endoscopic view of inflamed bladder.

Incidence
Up to 20% of women will have an attack in any one year.

Aetiology
1 *Escherichia coli* is the common infecting organism in 85% of cases.
2 *Staphylococcus epidermidis* and *Proteus mirabilis* in young, sexually active women.
3 Sexual activity increases incidence by 40 times.
4 Diaphragms and lubricated condoms.
5 Postmenopausal women with low Lactobacillus counts in the vagina.

Symptoms
1 Frequency of, and scalding pain on, micturition.

Bacterial cystitis

2 Dysuria.
3 Fishy smell to urine.
4 Suprapubic pain.
5 Urgency and strangury.
6 Malaise, fever and backache.

Management of the acute attack
1 Urine culture is not always necessary in GP's surgery. Midstream, clean catch of urine for blood and pus cells and culture and sensitivity.
2 Dip-sticks to detect pyuria, or the nitrite test if laboratory services are not available.
3 First-line therapy—nitrofurantoin, 50 mg three times daily for 3 days, is recommended as it gives the best antibiotic cover without encouraging resistant strains.
4 Single-dose therapy is also advocated as it increases patient compliance, induces less resistance and is cost-effective. Recommended regimens are:
    (a) trimethoprim, 600 mg stat.;
    (b) ciprofloxacin, 500 mg stat.;
    (c) cephalexin, 3 g stat.
Adjust when results of culture are known.

Special points

1 Pus cells in the urine in the absence of organisms may indicate chlamydial infection.
2 If pregnant, diabetic or suspect underlying cause Rx 7/7 penicillin or cephalosporin. Monitor closely for relapse.

Bacterial cystitis

Recurrent bacterial cystitis

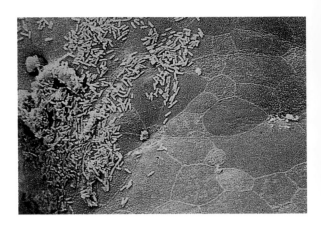

Fig 10.2 Scanning electron micrograph showing *Escherichia coli* adhering to bladder mucosa. With permission.

Aetiology

Usually reinfection with *E. coli* and associated with the following.

1 Incomplete emptying.
2 Low fluid intake.
3 Sexual intercourse with trauma to urethra.
4 80% of long-stay or debilitated patients with dementia and incontinence.

Management

1 Repeat urine culture if possible to confirm reinfections.
2 General advice:
    (a) high fluid intake to flush bladder;
    (b) void early after sexual intercourse;
    (c) care with perineal hygiene;
    (d) oestrogen therapy in postmenopausal women to increase colonisation with Lactobacillus and reduce vaginal pH.
3 Short, 3-day courses of antibiotics:
    (a) trimethoprim, 200 mg twice daily for 3 days;

Bacterial cystitis

(b) nitrofurantoin, 50 mg four times daily for 3 days;

(c) norfloxacin, 400 mg twice daily for 3 days;

(d) cephalexin, 250 mg four times daily for 3 days.

4 For sexually related infections, single-dose therapy taken postcoitally can be helpful. The bladder should be emptied after sexual intercourse and the perineum washed.

5 For frequent infections, institute long-term, low-dose prophylactic therapy:

(a) nitrofurantoin, 100 mg *nocte* for 3–6 months;

(b) norfloxacin, 400 mg twice daily for 3 months;

(c) Hexamine hippurate, 1 g twice daily for 3 months.

6 Refer for further investigation if the patient has:

(a) symptoms that are recurrent and unresponsive to treatment;

(b) fever;

(c) persistent haematuria;

(d) acute pyelonephritis and loin pain;

(e) children with urinary infections.

7 Investigations will include:

(a) plain X-ray of abdomen;

(b) ultrasound of kidney and bladder for residual urine;

(c) intravenous pyelography.

8 Refer for cystoscopy if:

(a) persistent haematuria;

(b) older women with recurrent or nonresponsive symptoms;

Special points

Young women with chlamydial infection may present with dysuria and frequency. Check and screen partner as well.

Bacterial cystitis

(c) pathology on imaging;
(d) constant bladder discomfort and sensory disorders.

Non-bacterial cystitis or interstitial cystitis

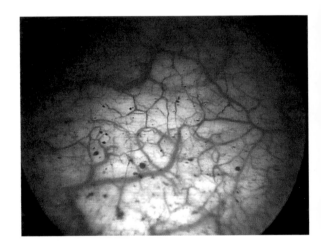

Fig 10.3 The fragile, bleeding urothelium after filling and emptying.

Aetiology
1 Could be defect in the bladder wall allowing urine to leak in to cause a pancystitis with intense lymphocyte and mast cell infiltration.
2 May be autoimmune.

Symptoms
1 Constant awareness of bladder.
2 Feeling of incomplete emptying.

Non-bacterial cystitis or interstitial cystitis

3 Frequency and dependency on toilet availability.
4 Nocturnal frequency and waking.
5 Often given frequent courses of antibiotics by GP in an attempt to treat it.
6 May be self-treated for 'thrush'.
7 Miserable and anxious, with recurrent or constant symptoms.
8 Social and sexual problems may develop.

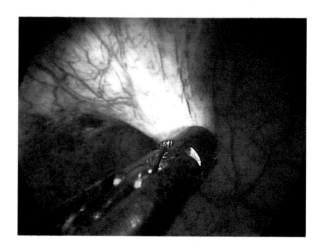

Fig 10.4 Bladder wall biopsy.

Diagnosis
1 Urine culture is usually negative for bacteria.
2 A volume and frequency chart of micturition kept over periods of 24 h is helpful to diagnose sensory disorders and micturition pattern.
3 Urodynamics may help to exclude detrusor instability.
4 Cystoscopy and bladder wall biopsies.
   (a) Allow assessment of bladder neck,

Non-bacterial cystitis or interstitial cystitis

volume capacity and urothelium. Vascular fragility and petechial haemorrhages on second fill of bladder are useful diagnostic pointers to interstitial cystitis.

(b) Mast cells on histology may be helpful in the diagnosis.

(c) Malignancy in older women can be excluded.

Management

1 Advise to:

(a) maintain a high fluid intake;

(b) avoid tea and coffee;

(c) maintain good introital hygiene and no sprays or deodorants;

(d) void early after sexual intercourse.

2 Institute bladder drill—holding longer between voids to build up to 2–2.5 h if possible.

3 Raise urinary pH. Effercitrate sachets may be helpful on a short-term basis.

4 Drug therapy. No protocol has yet received universal approval but:

(a) prolonged prophylactic antibiotic therapy, e.g. nitrofurantoin, is often given.

(b) bladder relaxation at night to promote sleep—imipramine, 50 mg *nocte*;

(c) small doses of steroids, e.g. prednisolone, 10 mg daily for 3 months, have been advocated;

(d) biofeedback to increase bladder control has been used.

Special points

With a lot of help and encouragement, many patients recover from this condition, but may need several intermittent courses of therapy.

Recurrent cystitis in postmenopausal women

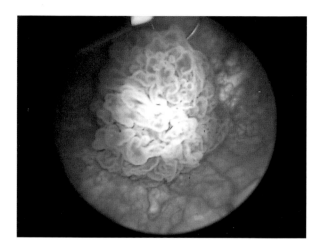

Fig 10.5 Endoscopic view of bladder carcinoma in older woman with haematuria and recurrent dysuria.

Aetiology

Lactobacillus competes with *E. coli* for epithelial receptor sites so that, after the menopause, when oestrogen levels fall, lactobacilli disappear and urogenital atrophy predisposes to urinary infections.

Symptoms

Recurrent cystitis in postmenopausal women should initiate further investigation as the incidence of pelvic pathology is higher.

Investigations

1 Should have urine checked for red cells.
2 Should receive vaginal oestriol.
3 Should have a pelvic examination with ultrasound and early referral for cystoscopy and biopsy to exclude polyps or malignancy.

Genuine stress incontinence (GSI)

The commonest form of incontinence, involving the involuntary loss of urine leading to social and hygiene problems.

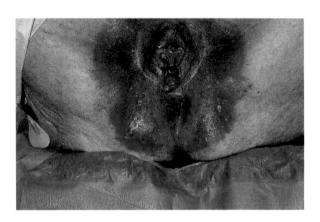

Fig 10.6 An 80-year-old widow with long-standing incontinence and ammonia dermatitis.

Incidence
10% of women are affected enough to consider their leakage to be a social or hygiene problem.

Aetiology
Urine leaks with the following.
1 Coughing, sneezing and exercise, e.g. aerobics.
2 Congenital weakness exhibited by some women.
3 Pregnancy—increased abdominal pressure.
4 Obesity.
5 Pelvic laxity following vaginal deliveries and pelvic floor trauma.
6 The menopause.

Genuine stress incontinence (GSI)

Symptoms

1 Embarrassing leakage of urine.
2 Frequency of micturition to prevent incontinence.
3 Poor flow and incomplete emptying if associated with prolapse.

Diagnosis

1 Check for leakage in the dorsal lithotomy position.
2 Examine for prolapse.
3 Check for abdominal masses.
4 Elderly—perform a rectal examination to exclude faecal impaction.
5 Saddle area—neurological check.
6 Urodynamics will be arranged by a specialist clinic if surgery is contemplated.

General measures and advice for mild cases or infirm patients

1 Exclude a urinary infection and check for glycosuria and haematuria. If haematuria is present, refer for cystoscopy.
2 Reduce diuretics in the elderly if possible.
3 Restrict fluid intake in the evenings and advise to avoid tea, coffee and alcohol.
4 Reduce weight in obese women if possible.
5 Constipation must be treated and smoking avoided, especially if chronic cough is present.
6 Postmenopausal women should be offered hormone replacement therapy (HRT) to reduce irritative urinary symptoms either systemically or locally.

Special points

Advances in sanitary protection have occurred, and patients need advice from a continence nurse or adviser on suitable protection. This increases confidence.

Genuine stress incontinence (GSI)

7 Diabetics must aim for a good control of blood sugar.

Management of GSI
Depends on age, fitness and commitment.

Physiotherapy
Physiotherapists interested in stress incontinence can help up to 70% of committed patients to improve.
1 Pelvic floor exercises.
2 Electrical stimulation.
3 Vaginal cones.

Mechanical devices
Most are still under review and all lead to abrasions or infections, but may help long-term cases.

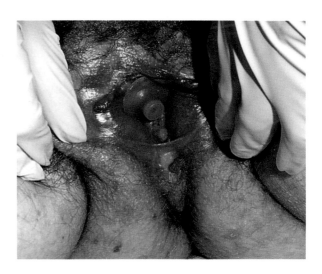

Fig 10.7 Urethral device *in situ.*

Genuine stress incontinence (GSI)

1 Tampons.
2 Urethral plugs.
3 Vaginal devices.
4 Intraurethral devices.

Surgery
Aims to elevate the bladder neck and reposition the proximal urethra intra-abdominally.
1 Anterior colporrhaphy — good for prolapse but not stress incontinence. Low success rate. No longer recommended.
2 Burch colposuspension — good for prolapse and stress incontinence. The best choice.
  (a) Cure rates: 95% at 1 year; 85% at 5 years; 70% at 10–12 years.
  (b) 12% of patients may have voiding difficulties afterwards.
  (c) Detrusor instability may arise in 17% of patients.
  (d) Rectocele may develop in 13% of patients within 5 years.
  (e) Can be performed laparoscopically.

Collagen urethral injections
1 Frail, elderly women with failed continence surgery may benefit from these bulking injections.
2 Day-case procedure under local anaesthetic.
3 Can be expensive.
4 Objective cure rate is 50% at 24 months.

Special points

1 Elderly women who get up at night should have a night light to prevent falls and injury.
2 Frequency may be better handled with a commode placed near the bed.
3 The insertion of a tampon before exercise may keep young women continent.

Detrusor instability

This is the second commonest cause of incontinence.

Incidence
1 10% of women experience this 'urge incontinence.'
2 Common in young children and causes nocturnal enuresis.
3 30% of women over 70 years of age have it.
4 Incontinence may occur during sexual intercourse.

Aetiology
1 The bladder contracts spontaneously or on provocation, e.g. filling.
2 Overexcitability of the detrusor muscle cells and reduced motor innervation of the bladder wall have been cited.

Symptoms
1 Severe daytime frequency.
2 Uncontrollable leakage of urine in response to a variety of stimulants, e.g. running water, returning home and placing 'key in the door'.
3 Exacerbations and remissions.
4 Nocturia.
5 Urgency and urge incontinence.

Diagnosis
1 Volume and frequency chart.
2 Urodynamics.
3 Midstream urine (MSU) to exclude infection and urine cytology.
4 Straight abdominal X-ray to exclude bladder stones and renal ultrasound.

Detrusor instability

Management

To re-establish central control, the following can be used.

1 Bladder drill—the patient has to void at set intervals: 60–90 min initially, increasing the interval slowly over a few weeks.

2 Biofeedback—more readily available now and aims to increase patient awareness of her bladder contractions.

3 Anticholinergic drugs, e.g. oxybutynin, 2.5 mg twice or three times daily, or can be used speculatively or prophylactically by the patient. Side effects of a dry mouth and blurring of vision can be troublesome. Tolterodine tartrate, 2 mg twice daily may produce less side effects. Propantheline, 15–30 mg three times daily before meals, is an alternative therapy especially for frequency.

4 Imipramine, 50 mg *nocte,* is useful for women with nocturnal enuresis.

5 Oestrogen—postmenopausal women may benefit from local or systemic oestrogen.

Surgery

1 Rarely advocated.

2 Bladder enlargement with a loop of ileum—Clam enterocystoplasty.

Special points

1 A continence adviser is an invaluable member of the team and can advise on general measures and sanitary protection, as well as performing assessments in the patient's home.
2 Cure rates are poor and there is a high placebo effect on all treatments for detrusor instability.

Detrusor instability

National organisations
1 The Continence Foundation, The Basement, 2 Doughty Street, London, WC1N 2PH. Telephone: 0171 404 6875.
2 Association for Continence Advice, Winchester House, Kennington Park, London, SW9 6EJ. Telephone: 0171 820 8113.
3 InconTact (National Association on Incontinence), 4 St Pancras Way, London, NW1 0PE. Telephone: 0171 831 9831.
4 ERIC (Enuresis Resource Information Centre), 65 St Michael's Hill, Bristol, BS2 8DZ. Telephone: 0117 926 4920.

11 Hormone replacement therapy (HRT) and osteoporosis

Hormone replacement therapy (HRT)

The mean age of the menopause in the UK is 50.8 years and the life expectancy of the female population is 82 years.

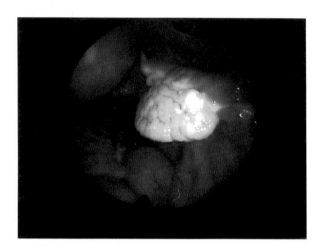

Fig 11.1 The shrivelled, menopausal ovary.

Reasons for prescribing HRT

1 Control of short-term symptoms:
  (a) vasomotor flushes and sweats;
  (b) vaginal dryness and dyspareunia;
  (c) insomnia and emotional lability;
  (d) dysuria and urinary frequency.

2 Management of surgically induced or premature menopause.

3 Prophylaxis against long-term sequelae of oestrogen deficiency, including:
  (a) osteoporosis and hip fractures — 50% reduction in incidence if HRT given for 5 years;
  (b) cardiovascular disease — heart disease is the principal cause of death in women over 45

Hormone replacement therapy (HRT)

years of age. There may be a protective effect on the cardiovascular system in the long term with increased survival after myocardial infarction.

4 Control of heavy, erratic, dysfunctional bleeding in perimenopausal women with anaemia who do not wish to have a hysterectomy.

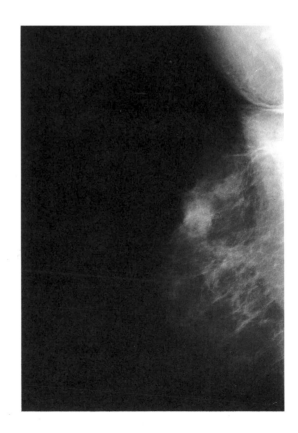

Fig 11.2 Mammography of early carcinoma of the breast—note calcification.

Hormone replacement therapy (HRT)

Contraindications to HRT

1 Carcinoma of the breast, unless patient and breast surgeon request because of severe menopausal symptoms.

2 Carcinoma of the endometrium — may be used if the disease has been eradicated.

3 Undiagnosed vaginal bleeding.

4 Active deep vein thrombosis (DVT), thromboembolic disorders or a history of confirmed venous thrombosis.

HRT is not contraindicated in the following conditions and can be safely used

1 Ischaemic heart disease and hypertension.

2 Varicose veins.

3 Benign breast disorders.

4 Uterine fibroids.

5 Carcinoma of the ovary.

6 Abnormal cervical smears.

7 Migraine.

8 Smoking.

9 Diabetes.

10 Malignant melanoma.

11 Raised cholesterol and triglycerides.

12 Epilepsy.

13 Planned surgery — do not stop medication before, unless very long procedure or prolonged bed rest anticipated.

14 Long-term anticoagulation.

15 Endometriosis.

Special points

Women with a history of breast cysts and mastalgia or breast cancer in the family are particularly concerned about taking HRT, and can be reassured about its safety in benign breast disorders.

Hormone replacement therapy (HRT)

Counselling for HRT

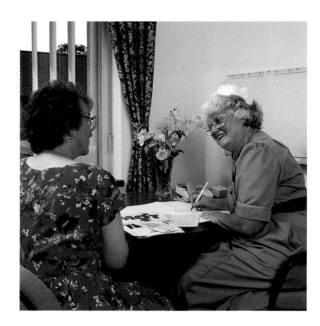

Fig 11.3 A positive approach should be adopted when counselling women about HRT.

Special points

Specific questions about a family history of thromboembolic episodes must be asked. A thrombophilia screen may be needed.

Lifestyle

1 Women should be advised to follow a low-fat, high-fibre diet as weight gain is common and can be distressing at this time.

2 Overweight women should be supervised to reduce weight actively.

3 Smokers should be strongly advised and supported to give up the habit.

4 Alcohol consumption and weekly limits should be discussed.

5 Regular weekly exercise, e.g. walking, is important.

Hormone replacement therapy (HRT)

Contraception

1 Ovulation can occur right up to the menopause.

2 HRT is *not* a contraceptive.

3 Barrier methods should be used for:

(a) 2 years after periods cease in women under 50 years of age;

(b) 1 year after periods cease in women over 50 years of age.

Special points

It is important to ask the women if she wants HRT. No woman should be coerced into having HRT and some will change their minds after the consultation and fail to obtain the prescription. Only one-third of users continue beyond 12 months.

Depression, anxiety and psychiatric symptoms

1 These need to be noted and managed with counselling and drug therapy if necessary.

2 Many women are only asking for advice and reassurance that what they are experiencing has no sinister cause.

Prophylactic aspect

1 Long-term benefits of HRT need to be emphasised, especially cardiovascular and osteoporosis protection.

2 Support is needed if minor side effects develop, otherwise a high drop out rate will occur.

Special points

The experiences of friends taking HRT can strongly influence the decision of the individual woman.

Hormone replacement therapy (HRT)

Patient fears — women with contraindications must be excluded

Only 15% of eligible women use HRT.

1 Breast cancer is the greatest fear. Teach breast awareness and advise participation in National Mammography Screening (see advice on p. 221).

2 Weight gain (see advice on p. 227).

3 Continuation of menstrual periods — probably main reason for giving up especially if heavy or painful (see advice on p. 216 about period-free regimens).

4 Premenstrual symptoms (see advice on p. 224).

5 Belief that it is unnatural:
  (a) they do not like taking 'pills';
  (b) they are putting off the 'inevitable';
  (c) the symptoms will recur when medication ceases;
  (d) many women support homeopathy and complementary therapies in preference to conventional therapies.

Diagnosis

Clinical symptoms

1 Vasomotor symptoms and vaginal dryness are the most reliable pointers;

2 amenorrhoea of more than 6 months' duration (only 10% will menstruate again).

Biochemical investigations

1 Serum oestradiol — of limited value;

Special points

Many thousands of women worldwide have had miserable menopausal symptoms alleviated and the quality of their lives enhanced by HRT.

Hormone replacement therapy (HRT)

2 follicle-stimulating hormone (FSH) — useful in:

(a) amenorrhoeic women and in those still menstruating if over 30 U/l;

(b) premature menopause — symptoms before aged 40 years; two or three persistently raised levels (>30 U/l);

(c) women on the oral contraceptive pill: perimenopausal women on the combined oral contraceptive pill (COCP) can stop the COCP and have an FSH level taken 8 weeks later to determine menopausal status; peri-menopausal women on the progestogen-only pill do not need to stop, and a raised FSH on two occasions would suggest ovarian failure.

Important target group

Women who have undergone a hysterectomy before 45 years of age with ovarian conservation may have an earlier menopause, and FSH levels should be checked to detect ovarian failure every few years.

Secial points

In view of the small increase in breast cancer after 8–10 years of therapy, it is important to commence HRT when needed and not prematurely for other reasons.

Hormone replacement therapy (HRT)

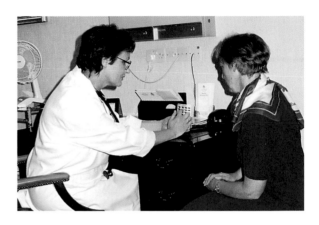

Fig 11.4 Getting off to a good start.

Initial examination

1 General examination with reference to blood pressure, cardiovascular state and breast examination. Mammography if indicated.

2 Cervical smear and note if hysterectomy has been performed. If so, enquire about oophorectomy.

3 Pelvic examination to exclude fibroids.

4 Metabolic disorders and thyroid disease need to be diagnosed, but are unusual.

5 Blood tests. Full blood count (FBC) and FSH if indicated.

Side effects are usually of a minor nature

1 Return of menstruation with some preparations. This is usually acceptable to most women. Period-free regimens used for those 'not keen on periods'.

2 Nausea and breast tenderness—subside with usage.

Hormone replacement therapy (HRT)

3 Leg cramps and limb pains — not related to venous thrombosis.
4 Premenstrual tension (PMT) symptoms.

Starting treatment
1 Realistic expectations — HRT is not a panacea for youth.
2 Different preparations may need to be tried as different progestogens suit different women.
3 Effective symptom control — may take 3 months to achieve. Use a menstrual calendar to record and assess.
4 If symptoms persist, increase to a maximum dose. In non-responders, consider other causes of symptoms, e.g. thyroid disease, alcohol excess and depression.

Management
1 Preparations can be selected according to the patient's age and symptoms (see Table 11.1).
2 Oestrogen, the beneficial HRT hormone, is available as vaginal pessaries, oral tablets, patches, skin gels and subcutaneous implants.
3 Progesterone is added to control endometrial stimulation, and is available orally and by patch therapy. Progestogen-only creams are on trial at present to evaluate their effectiveness.

Special points

A 3-month 'trial of HRT' can be given to women with intermittent or equivocal symptoms and therapy continued if a good response is reported.

Special points

There is no perceived benefit in giving women who have had a hysterectomy a progestogen.

HRT for the older woman

The vagina becomes drier, thinner and shrinks after the menopause.

Hormone replacement therapy (HRT)

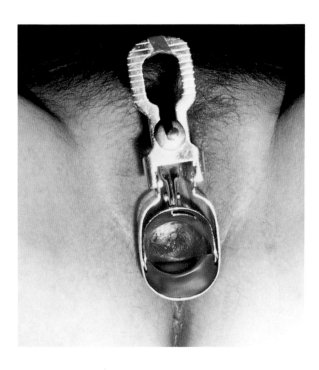

Fig 11.5 Atrophic vaginitis.

Table 11.1 Choice of medication.

Patient	Symptom	Choice of medication
Older woman	Vaginal dryness only	Local oestrogen
Post-hysterectomy	Symtoms	Oestrogen only required
Woman with intact uterus:		
premenopausal	Symptoms + regular periods	Monthly cyclical HRT (see p. 214)
perimenopausal	Symptoms + patchy amenorrhoea	Monthly cyclical HRT (see p. 214) or quarterly bleed HRT (see p. 215)
postmenopausal	Symptoms + prolonged (12 months) amenorrhoea or over 54 years of age	Continuous combined HRT or tibolone

Hormone replacement therapy (HRT)

Medication

Local oestrogen treatment used to alleviate atrophic vaginitis, vaginal dryness and dyspareunia.

1 The older woman with few vasomotor symptoms, but sexually active and experiencing vaginal dryness, dyspareunia and periurethral irritation.

2 Women wearing ring pessaries for prolapse control. Local oestrogen thickens the vaginal epithelium and encourages lactobacilli and a better vaginal pH.

3 Preoperatively can be used to improve tissue before vaginal surgery.

Special points

1 Oestrogen cream can be absorbed systemically and this limits the duration of use.

2 Recommmended: Ortho-Gynest® pessaries — oestriol and less absorption.

Drug	Oestrogen delivery
Ovestin®	Cream
Ortho-Gynest®	Pessaries
Vagifem®	Pessaries
Estring®	Vaginal ring
Replens®	Non-hormonal

Hormone replacement therapy (HRT)

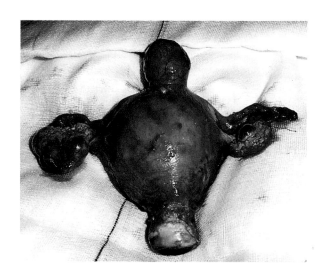

Fig 11.6 Hysterectomy performed for cysts and fibroid.

HRT post-hysterectomy

Twenty per cent of British women undergo hysterectomy for gynaecological problems.

Medication

Oral therapy
1 There is no need for progestogen.
2 Start with oral therapy as it is safe, well-proven, inexpensive and has a long-term benefit.

Drug	Oestrogen	Dose
Premarin®	Conjugated oestrogen	0.625 or 1.25 mg
Climaval®	Oestradiol valerate	1 or 2 mg
Zumenon®	Oestradiol	1 or 2 mg
Progynova®	Oestradiol valerate	1 or 2 mg
Elleste-Solo®	Oestradiol valerate	1 or 2 mg

Hormone replacement therapy (HRT)

3 Allow a 3-month trial of oral therapy and increase the dose if necessary before suggesting a change. If there is incomplete resolution of symptoms, proceed to oestrogen patch therapy with a *matrix* patch (see below).

Patch therapy
1 If there is incomplete resolution of symptoms, e.g. hot flushes, on oral therapy, proceed to patch therapy which provides transdermal oestrogen; 37.5, 40 or 50 μg is a good dose to start with and can be adjusted up or down.
2 The matrix patch causes less skin irritation than the reservoir patch. It is slim and discreet.
3 Patches should be changed twice a week.

Drug	Oestrogen	Dose
Evorel®	Transdermal	25–100 μg/24 h
Estraderm MX®	Transdermal	25–100 μg/24 h
Fematrix®	Transdermal	40 or 80 μg/24 h
Menorest®	Transdermal	37.5–75 μg/24 h
Dermestril®	Transdermal	25–100 μg/24 h

4 It may be easier for women to change patches once a week and, if preferred, the following could be prescribed.

Hormone replacement therapy (HRT)

Drug	Oestrogen	Dose
FemSeven®	Transdermal, releases oestradiol	50 µg daily
Progynova® TS	Transdermal, releases oestradiol	50 or 100 µg daily

5 Patch therapy is twice as expensive as oral therapy.

Special points

Oestrogen from adrenal precursors is produced in peripheral fatty tissue, so that obese women tend to be better oestrogenised and report fewer symptoms

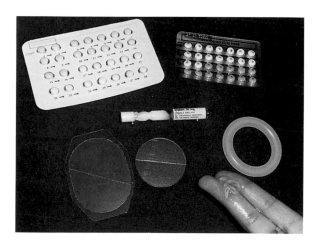

Fig 11.7 Oestrogen can be delivered by tablets, patches, rings, implants and gel.

Hormone replacement therapy (HRT)

The premenopausal woman

Medication

Oral and patch therapy

1 Women under 50 years of age with symptoms of the menopause, but regular periods, should commence oral sequential therapy to allow a monthly bleed and protect the endometrium.

Drug	Oestrogen/dose	Progestogen/dose
Prempak-C®	Conjugated oestrogen/0.625 or 1.2 mg	Norgestrel/150 μg
Climagest®	Oestradiol valerate/1 or 2 mg	Norethisterone/1 mg
Nuvelle®	Oestradiol valerate/2 mg	Levonorgestrel/75 μg
Femoston®	Oestradiol/1 or 2 mg	Dydrogesterone/10 mg
Elleste-Duet®	Oestradiol/2 mg	Norethisterone/1 mg
Premique® Cycle	Conjugated oestrogen/0.625 mg	Medroxyprogesterone acetate/10 mg

2 Incomplete response to oral therapy. Proceed to patch therapy with:

  (a) an oestrogen matrix patch with added progestogen tablets to induce bleeding;

Drug	Oestrogen/dose	Progestogen/dose
Evorel® Pak	Oestradiol/50 μg	Norethisterone/1 mg
Estrapak®	Oestradiol/50 μg	Norethisterone/1 mg
Femapak®	Oestradiol/40 or 80 μg	Dydrogesterone/10 mg

Hormone replacement therapy (HRT)

(b) a sequential patch containing oestrogen and a progestogen.

Drug	Oestrogen/dose	Progestogen/dose
Nuvelle® /TS	Oestradiol/80 µg plus	Levonorgestrel/20 µg
Evorel® /Sequi	Oestradiol/50 µg plus	Norethisterone/170 µg

The perimenopausal woman

Medication

Oral and patch therapy

1 Women aged 50–54 years experiencing symptoms of the menopause and erratic menstrual cycles could be given oral sequential therapy to induce monthly bleeds or sequential patch therapy (as described above).

2 They may prefer three-monthly or quarterly bleeds with a long oestrogen phase and a 14-day progestogen phase to induce endometrial shedding.

3 Lower endogenous oestrogen levels in this age group will allow three-monthly manipulation of the bleed phase.

Special points

Breakthrough bleeding on Tridestra® indicates the need to return to shorter cycle induced bleeds.

Drug	Oestrogen/dose	Progestogen/dose
Tridestra®	Oestradiol/2 mg	Medroxyprogesterone/20 mg for 14 days

Hormone replacement therapy (HRT)

The postmenopausal woman

Medication

Oral therapy

1 After the age of 54 years, 90% of women are amenorrhoeic and in the postmenopausal state.

2 Resumption of periods can be unwelcome as these may be painful and heavy.

3 Period-free regimens should be selected at this age. These regimens are not 'bleed free' — up to 50% of women may spot during the first 6 months and need to be warned to expect this.

4 Oral continuous combined therapy will induce and keep the endometrium in a near-atrophic state.

Drug	Oestrogen/dose	Progestogen/dose
Premique®	Conjugated oestrogen/0.625 mg	Medroxyprogesterone/5 mg
Climesse®	Oestradiol/2 mg	Norethisterone/0.7 mg
Kliofem®	Oestradiol/2 mg	Norethisterone/1 mg

5 Tibolone (Livial®) is a useful drug for the older woman with an intact uterus. A synthetic steroid, licensed for osteoporosis prevention, it can be used if PMT or oestrogenic side effects, such as headaches and breast tenderness develop on other formulations. Initial spotting should give way to amenorrhoea. A mood elevating effect is described. May increase libido.

Hormone replacement therapy (HRT)

Drug	Action	Dose
Livial®	Gonadomimetic	2.5 mg daily

Patch therapy
Patch therapy is an alternative and a new product is available.

Drug	Oestrogen/dose	Progestogen/dose
Evorel®/Conti	Oestradiol/50 µg	Norethisterone/170 µg daily

Other oestrogen delivery systems

Gels
Oestradiol delivered daily, transdermally, by gel application is attractive to some women.

Drug	Oestrogen	Dose
Oestrogel®	Oestradiol	1.5 mg
Sandrena®	Oestradiol	0.5 or 1 mg daily

Implants
1 Subcutaneously inserted oestradiol implants

Hormone replacement therapy (HRT)

of three different strengths give symptom relief for 5–8 months.

2 Easy insertion as an office procedure and well liked by patients.

3 Fatigue and low libido can be helped by the simultaneous insertion of a testosterone 100-mg implant.

4 Serum oestradiol measurements prior to further implants can be helpful in preventing tachyphylaxis.

Selective oestrogen receptor modulators (SERMs)

1 Raloxifene, a non-steroidal benzothiophene, modulates oestrogen receptors selectively.

2 Women on conventional HRT have to be warned about the slight increased incidence of breast cancer and, for many, endometrial stimulation and the return of bleeding are unwelcome.

3 There is a need for a new drug to repress morbidity from cardiovascular and osteoporotic disease in postmenopausal women.

4 Raloxifene called EVISTA® is available on the UK market now for the prevention of osteoporosis and the initial trial showed that it:

(a) improves postmenopausal lipid profiles (total and low-density lipoprotein (LDL) cholesterol);

(b) improves bone mineral density — regionally and totally;

(c) has no adverse effects on endometrial or breast tissue.

5 The drawback is that hot flushes are not

> **Special points**
>
> Both gels and implants should be administered with a progestogen to induce endometrial shedding in women with an intact uterus.

Hormone replacement therapy (HRT)

improved and, although the results are encouraging, more data will need to be accumulated.

Follow-up on patients
1 See in 3 months to check blood pressure. Occasional patient has an idiosyncratic rise in blood pressure.

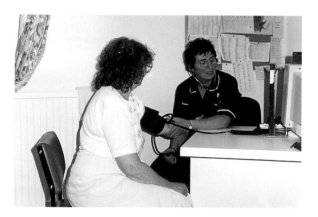

Fig 11.8 Follow-up.

2 Confirm normal withdrawal bleeding pattern if appropriate, discuss any concerns and assess minor side effects.
3 Patients should be seen at 6-monthly to yearly intervals thereafter.
4 Practice nurses trained in menopause supervision have a major role as women often consult them first or at smear taking.
5 Good patient information is essential and many drug companies have such material for distribution.

Hormone replacement therapy (HRT)

Special points

1 Postmenopausal women are not completely oestrogen deficient.

2 About one-third is produced in the hilar cells of the ovary and many women have few symptoms and feel well at this oestrogen level.

6 Gynaecological referral should be considered for women with the following symptoms after starting HRT:

(a) heavy, painful periods;

(b) frank bleeding after amenorrhoea on 'non-period' regimens;

(c) repetitive or heavy breakthrough bleeding;

(d) postcoital bleeding.

These women may have gynaecological pathology in the uterus which has been unmasked by the HRT.

Questions and answers about HRT

When should HRT be started?

1 As soon as vasomotor and urogenital symptoms develop in perimenopausal women. Menstrual cycles may still be regular.

2 At the time of hysterectomy and bilateral salpingo-oophorectomy.

3 Early advice to women who have had oestrogen deficiency states, e.g. anorexia nervosa, prolonged amenorrhoea.

Is HRT a contraceptive?

No, and advice on sterilisation, vasectomy or an intrauterine contraceptive device (IUD) or

Questions and answers about HRT

Mirena® intrauterine system (IUS) should be given.

When can HRT be stopped?
1 Review the situation at the age of 60 years or after 8–10 years of therapy.
2 Aim for 5 years of therapy to achieve best long-term physiological health.

Can an FSH level be used to diagnose the menopause?
1 It can be helpful if over 30 U/l.
2 Perimenopausal women may have oestrogen surges and fluctuating symptoms.
3 Reliance on clinical symptoms is recommended.

What advice should patients receive regarding breast cancer?
1 The short-term use (less than 5 years) is not associated with increased risk.
2 There is a 30% increased incidence of breast cancer with long-term use.
3 This excess risk is outweighed by a reduction in mortality from all causes and mortality from all cancers and even breast cancer.
4 Women who develop breast cancer whilst on HRT have a better prognosis for survival as they receive increased surveillance and have lower grade tumours than non-HRT users who develop cancer.
5 If there is a family history of breast cancer in first-degree relatives, the patient has an

Questions and answers about HRT

increased risk until the age of 60 years. HRT can be given, however, for short- to medium-term use with mammography.

What can be offered to women with breast cancer who develop menopausal symptoms?
1 Tamoxifen itself can be helpful, 20 mg daily.
2 Megestrol acetate, 40–80 mg daily.
3 Norethisterone, 10 mg daily.
4 Medroxyprogesterone acetate, 20 mg daily.
5 Short-term use of HRT may be safe and even provide some protection.
6 Women with benign breast disease are not at excess risk of developing breast cancer on HRT, and after assessment of a benign breast lump can restart HRT if desired. Livial® is recommended.

Hormone Replacement Therapy (HRT) and Breast Cancer Information for Patients

A comprehensive new report on hormone replacement therapy (HRT) and the development of breast cancer has just been published. This leaflet explains what the research shows and what it means for you.

The benefits of HRT
HRT is effective in relieving unpleasant symptoms of the menopause and, when taken for several years, prevents fractures which are caused by thinning of the bones (osteoporosis). It may also reduce heart disease.

Continued on p. 223

Questions and answers about HRT

HRT and breast cancer — the new research

For some time it has been thought possible that more cases of breast cancer are diagnosed in women who use HRT than in those who do not. The new research confirms this and also finds that those breast cancers found in women on HRT are easier to treat than those in women not on HRT. The chances of developing breast cancer are higher for those who use HRT for many years. Those who use it for a short period around the menopause are hardly affected.

For women aged 50 not using HRT, about 45 in every 1000 will have cancer diagnosed over the next 20 years, i.e. up to age 70. For those who use HRT for long periods of time, the estimated number of extra cancers is shown below:

Length of time on HRT	Extra breast cancers in HRT users, above the 45 occurring in non-users, over 20 years
5 years in use	2 per 1000
10 years in use	6 per 1000
15 years in use	12 per 1000

The extra chance of developing breast cancer on HRT does not persist beyond about 5 years after stopping treatment.

What to do if you are concerned

If you are on HRT this research does not mean that you need to stop taking it. If you are concerned and want to know more, you should make a routine non-urgent appointment with your doctor.

All women, and especially those on HRT, should be aware of any changes that occur in their breasts, and report them to their doctor. All women aged between 50 and 64 are invited to have regular, 3-yearly mammograms, and those 65 and over may have them on request.

Questions and answers about HRT

How is PMT on HRT handled?
1 Progestogenic side effects, such as bloating, irritability, mood swings and breast discomfort, can occur.
2 Change to a different progestogen, e.g. some women are better on dydrogesterone or medroxyprogesterone acetate.
3 Consider progesterone by a non-oral route.
4 Consider continuous combined HRT.
5 Consider Livial®.

Is obesity a contraindication to HRT?
No. But increases risk of a DVT.

Can smokers use HRT?
Yes.

Can a woman with fibroids use HRT?
1 Yes. They may slowly enlarge and can be monitored by pelvic ultrasonography annually or biannually.
2 Large fibroids may increase further in size and menorrhagia may develop.
3 The patient has a choice of stopping treatment or undergoing hysterectomy.

Can a woman with endometriosis take HRT?
1 Yes. Fear that HRT would stimulate the progression of endometriosis is not supported by the data.
2 Continuous combined therapy, e.g. Premique® or Livial®, may be better.

Questions and answers about HRT

Should women have a mammogram before starting HRT?
1 Not necessarily unless high level of anxiety.
2 All should be on the National Breast Screening Programme which commences at the age of 50 years.

What advice is given if the patient stops bleeding on HRT?
Reassure the woman that the endometrium is atrophic and that there is no cause for concern.

How are heavy withdrawal bleeds managed?
1 Can be initial response to therapy and will settle. Exclude pathology, e.g. fibroids, by scan.
2 Change to a different progestogen or a 3-monthly bleed regimen if appropriate.
3 Refer for gynaecological opinion if persists.

How are breakthrough bleeds (BTBs) managed?

On sequential therapy
1 Early cycle BTB indicates inadequate oestrogen—try a larger dose.
2 Late cycle bleeds—progestogen insufficient and should be changed or increased.

On continuous combined therapy
1 Often happens on 'period-free' regimens and must be investigated if persists for more than 6 months.
2 Persistent irregular bleeds need gynaecologi-

Questions and answers about HRT

cal referral for scan, endometrial sampling and hysteroscopy.

How can menstrual migraine be managed?
1 Migraines tend to occur premenstrually and during the first days of the bleed.
2 For perimenopausal women, try a small supplemental oestradiol 25-µg patch during the headache-susceptible time and check that a good withdrawal bleed occurs.
3 A drop in oestrogen level is the trigger, so transdermal or percutaneous oestrogen regimens can be tried for menstruating women and oestrogen implants for women who have had a hysterectomy.
4 If migraines continue, change the progestogen or use transdermal progestogen as sometimes the fluctuating progestogen is the culprit, e.g. Evorel® Conti (see p. 217).

Can HRT help depression?
1 Depression can be at its worst in the last few years before the menstrual cycles end.
2 Women often report increased PMT at this time.
3 A trial of oestrogen therapy can be given rather than psychoactive drugs and the response assessed.

How can continuance be encouraged?
1 Positive attitude on the part of the GP about the benefits of HRT.

Questions and answers about HRT

2 Good counselling on expectations and side effects, and fact sheet availability.
3 Easy access to nurse counsellor if problems arise.
4 Treat each woman and her approach to her problems as an individual.
5 If symptoms are incompletely resolved after 3 months of medication, check compliance, increase the oestrogen dosage or switch to patch therapy.

Does HRT cause weight gain?
1 Weight gain is a common occurrence in the middle years with an increase in total body fat.
2 There is no evidence from the current literature that HRT causes a gain in weight.
3 It can prevent the increase in male-type abdominal fat that accumulates after the menopause — the 'apple' shape.
4 A very small number of women may experience a sudden weight gain which disappears when oestrogens are discontinued.

Does HRT help prevent Alzheimer's disease?
1 Two studies report a benefit in oestrogen users with a lower incidence of Alzheimer's disease.
2 HRT given to established cases showed a benefit in mild to moderate dementia and decreased the risk of developing the condition.

Questions and answers about HRT

What are the risk factors for venous thrombosis to consider before prescribing HRT?

1 Obesity. Body mass index in excess of $30\,kg/m^2$.

2 Varicose veins. Only if surgery contemplated.

3 Superficial phlebitis. These women may be deficient in proteins C and S.

4 Family history. Congenital thrombophilia.

5 Personal history. Clear history of pulmonary embolism or proven DVT.

6 Surgery. Most departments institute prophylactic therapy.

7 Immobility.

8 Long haul air travel.

What is the risk of venous thromboembolism (VTE) on HRT?

1 There is an increase in the risk of VTE on HRT. The risk is very small, i.e. one case of VTE amongst 5000 women using HRT for 1 year, and is restricted to the first year of use.

2 The fatality rate is low and the occurrence of VTE is insignificant when weighed against the benefits of HRT on coronary heart disease and osteoporotic fractures.

3 Only 10% of cases of VTE will have underlying thrombophilia but, in women with congenital thrombophilia, oestrogen may act as an increased risk factor, as will immobility, surgery, obesity, age, medical conditions, etc.

Questions and answers about HRT

Advice to the patient

Past history of proven VTE and strong family history of thrombosis
1 Refer to haematologist for a screen for thrombophilia.
2 Avoid HRT if past severe episode, e.g. pulmonary embolism.
3 Avoid HRT if other ongoing risk factors.
4 Consider patch therapy.
5 Consider low-dose aspirin.

Proven cases of thrombophilia
1 Avoid HRT if previous VTE.
2 Avoid HRT if family history.

Hospital patients
1 Advise thromboprophylaxis (routine now).
2 For severe medical conditions, major surgery and prolonged bed rest, probably should stop HRT.
3 Before long haul flights, women on HRT could take half an aspirin.

Can HRT be prescribed for women with a previous DVT or pulmonary embolus?
1 If related to oral contraception or pregnancy state, do a clotting profile.
2 Antithrombin 3, protein C and protein S should be assayed. If normal, can take HRT.
3 Transdermal oestrogen preferred or Livial®.

Questions and answers about HRT

From the Committee on Safety of Medicines, Medicine Control Agency: Information on the risk of blood clots for women taking HRT

You may have read in the press or heard people discuss that women taking hormone replacement therapy (HRT) are prone to blood clots in their veins. The purpose of this leaflet is to explain the benefits and risks, and what this means for you.

The benefits of HRT

HRT relieves symptoms of the menopause and, when taken for several years, prevents fractures by reducing the thinning of the bones (osteoporosis). It has also been suggested that it may reduce heart disease.

The risk of a blood clot

New information was published in a medical journal in October 1996 which suggests that blood clots in the veins are more common in women who take HRT, whatever the type. However, the chance of getting a blood clot is low regardless of whether or not you take HRT. The risk is only during the first year of use.

Chances of getting a blood clot

Not taking HRT	1 in 10 000 per year
While taking HRT	3 in 10 000 per year

What are the consequences of a blood clot?

Blood clots can occur in any vein, but are most common in the legs (deep vein thrombosis or DVT) where they may cause pain, swelling or redness. If this occurs, patients may require certain tests and a few days' treatment in hospital. Occasionally, blood clots pass to the lungs; this is more serious, but usually responds to treatment.

How serious can a blood clot be?

Most people who get a blood clot in a vein make a complete

Continued on p. 231

Questions and answers about HRT

recovery after treatment, so the chance of dying from a blood clot is very low indeed. If you are not taking HRT, your chance of dying from a blood clot is 1 in a million per year: while you are taking HRT, your chance is 3 in a million per year.

What to do if you are concerned
The risk of blood clots is low and needs to be balanced against the benefits that HRT may have for you. If you are already on HRT, you do not need to stop it. If you are concerned about what you have heard or read and would like to discuss these concerns further, make a routine appointment to see your doctor who can talk you through the pros and cons of HRT with you.

How much supervision does the patient on HRT need?
Annual checks once established on a satisfactory regimen.

Questions and answers about HRT

Advice to women who do not want HRT

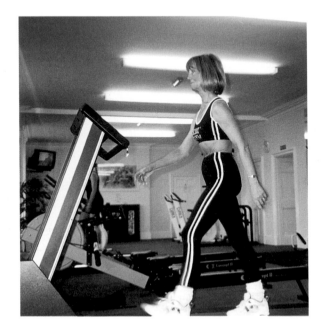

Fig 11.9 Grandmother taking regular exercise.

1 A healthy diet high in fibre and low in fat should be encouraged.
2 Regular weekly exercise should be under-taken, e.g. walking, swimming.
3 Alendronate and calcium supplements may prevent osteoporosis.
4 Clonidine for hot flushes has not proved to be helpful in the majority of women.
5 A period of rest during the day can be helpful if night sweats and insomnia are severe.
6 Sexual difficulties with vaginal dryness can be helped by water-soluble vaginal lubricants, e.g. Senselle®, Replens® (Lenipath), or local vaginal oestriol preparations.

Questions and answers about HRT

7 Complementary therapies, such as aroma-therapy and yoga, have become very popular in recent years. All focus on increasing a feeling of well-being and relaxation and decrease stress. Only specialist practitioners who are professionally accountable for the treatment should be recommended.

Special points

The menopause often coincides with other major life events, e.g. children leaving home, marital adjustments and care of elderly parents. These contribute further to stress and insomnia.

Osteoporosis

Osteoporosis is a skeletal disease that results in the reduction of the amount and strength of bone tissue.

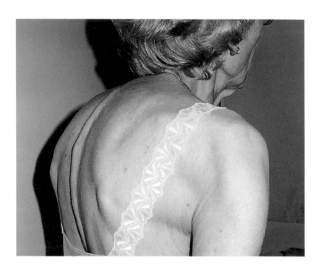

Fig 11.10 Note the 'Dowager's Hump'.

Incidence

1 One woman out of every two can expect to sustain an osteoporotic fracture by 70 years of age.

2 60% of elderly women experience vertebral wedging from osteoporosis, and 20% develop a crush fracture leading to loss of height and occasionally severe pain.

3 By the age of 70 years, 30% of bone mass may be lost. The loss is insidious and has been referred to as 'The Silent Epidemic'.

Aetiology

1 Women begin to lose bone at the menopause when oestrogen levels fall.

2 Immobility or lack of exercise in later years.

Osteoporosis

3 Suboptimal diet in teenage years and in older women.
4 Chronic ill health and steroid therapy.
5 Genetic propensity. Some women are 'fast bone losers'.

Diagnosis
1 The condition generally presents as a fracture, often following trivial trauma, e.g. slipping on ice.
2 Acute or recurrent backache and pelvic pain may suggest a vertebral crush fracture or femoral head osteoporosis.

Special points

1 There are huge socioeconomic costs of osteoporosis. Osteoporosis costs the UK National Health Service £750 million a year.
2 Significant quality of life issues are associated with osteoporosis. It is a common cause of pain, disability and death.

Prevention

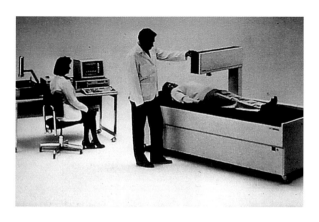

Fig 11.11 Dual-energy X-ray absorptiometry (DEXA) screening for selected cases. (With permission.)

Osteoporosis

The GP has a key role in identifying patients in the practice 'at risk' of osteoporosis, and in providing advice on diet and exercise in the long-term prevention of the condition.

Risk factors
1 Family history.
2 Slim Caucasian women.
3 Sedentary lifestyle.
4 Smoking.
5 High alcohol consumption.
6 Low parity and early menopause.
7 Steroid therapy.
8 Oestrogen deficiency states:
   (a) younger women: anorexic states, excessive exercise, premature menopause;
   (b) older women: menopause, immobilisation.

Screening
1 At risk patients should be sent for dual-energy X-ray absorptiometry (DEXA) to measure bone density.
2 Subsequent fracture risk can be predicted by comparing the patient with her peer group (more than 2.5 standard deviations below the mean suggests osteoporosis risk).
3 Population screening is not yet available and may not be cost-effective.

Osteoporosis

Treatment

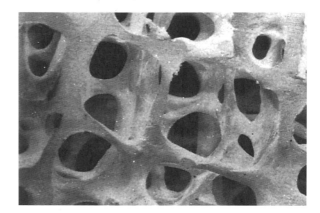

Fig 11.12 Healthy bone structure.

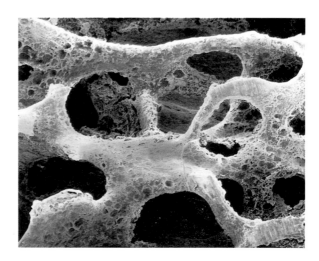

Fig 11.13 Osteoporotic bone structure. With permission from Professor P. Motta, Department of Anatomy, University 'La Sapienza', Rome. Science Photo Library.

1 A good diet adequate in calcium and vitamin D. Dairy products and vegetables are good sources of calcium, and low-fat products are readily available.

2 A reasonable amount of weekly exercise.

Osteoporosis

3 Avoidance of smoking and excessive alcohol consumption.

4 Bisphosphonates—alendronate (Fosamax®); 10 mg daily may be helpful in older women and osteoporotic patients, and is taken 30 min before meals and in a sitting position.

5 The 'gold standard' of care for the older woman is oestrogen replacement therapy. This reduces the incidence of fractures by 50% and prevents bone loss. Period-free regimens increase compliance in older women.

6 The British Menopause Society recommends the following therapeutic choices to achieve a serum oestradiol level above 150 pmol/l:

(a) conjugated equine oestrogens—0.625 mg (higher doses may be necessary for younger women with premature menopause);

(b) oestradiol (oral)—2 mg;

(c) oestradiol (transdermal)—50 μg;

(d) oestradiol (gel)—5 g (= 2 mg);

(e) oestradiol (implant)—50 mg (6-monthly);

(f) tibolone—2.5 mg.

Recommended HRT products

1 Period-free regimens—preferred as better results, e.g. Premique® or Climesse®.

2 Monthly bleed regimens, e.g. Prempak® or Nuvelle®.

3 Patch therapy, e.g. FemSeven® or Estraderm®.

4 Synthetic steroid, e.g. tibolone.

Management of osteoporotic fractures

1 Pain relief with non-opiate analgesics.

Special points

Young women should be encouraged to eat a balanced, healthy diet and to take regular exercise in order to lay down the maximum bone mass which is completed by the end of the third decade of life.

Special points

HRT is the treatment of choice to prevent osteoporosis.

Osteoporosis

2 Early mobilisation—avoid bed rest.
3 Physiotherapy.
4 Calcitonin may have a role.
5 Multidisciplinary team and post discharge support for hip replacement surgery.
6 Standard fracture management is difficult in elderly women, as the following can occur:
    (a) delay in bony union;
    (b) residual joint stiffness;
    (c) mental and physical frailty;
    (d) coexisting medical conditions;
    (e) loss of prefracture independence.

Summary

1 The preservation of bone mass remains the mainstay of treatment.
2 HRT is the best available intervention of proven benefit.
3 HRT can be used for 8–10 years.
4 Bisphosphonates could be introduced for 3 years in later years.
5 In the sixth and seventh decades, calcium and vitamin D can be used.

12 Hirsutism

Idiopathic hirsutism

The most commonly made diagnosis in women with excess facial and body hair.

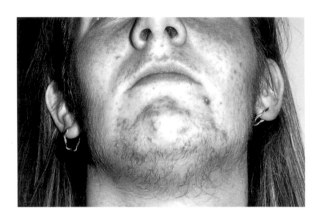

Fig 12.1 A 15-year-old school girl with hirsutism and acne.

Incidence
1 True hirsutism affects 10% of women, but almost 40% of Caucasian women consider that they have superfluous body hair and a large cosmetic industry caters for hair removal.
2 Women of Mediterranean and Indian origin have fine, dark facial hair which is a racial characteristic.

Aetiology
1 Increased circulating androgens or excessively responsive hair follicles.
2 Some women with iron deficiency anaemia and hypothyroidism may present with alopecia and hirsutism respectively.

Investigation
1 Serum testosterone concentration — if over 6 nmol/l, refer for specialist assessment as sug-

Idiopathic hirsutism

gests virilising tumour of ovary or adrenal gland.

2 Follicle-stimulating hormone (FSH) and luteinising hormone (LH) assay between Day 4 and Day 6 of cycle. LH of more than 10 IU/l suggests polycystic ovarian disorder.

3 Thyroid function test, thyroid-stimulating hormone (TSH), to diagnose hypothyroidism.

4 Serum ferritin if alopecia exists.

5 Transvaginal ultrasonography of ovaries.

Symptoms

Women with idiopathic hirsutism have the following.

1 Normal menstrual cycles.

2 Gradual onset of hirsutism after puberty.

3 Normal scalp hair.

4 Serum testosterone under 5 nmol/l.

5 Normal LH.

6 Facial, chest, breast and abdominal hair.

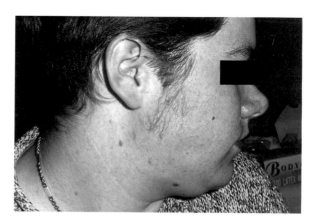

Fig 12.2 Facial hair and needs to shave chin daily.

Idiopathic hirsutism

Management

Control of hirsutism can be achieved by the following.

1 Local cosmetic treatments—depilation, waxing, shaving and electrolysis. These treatments do not encourage increased hair growth. They are expensive and time consuming. The role of laser treatment remains to be defined.

2 Explanation and reassurance may be all that is required. The condition has considerable psychological impact. Hair on the chest and back is considered to be repulsive by most women.

3 Combined oral contraceptive pill (COCP)— good first choice.

4 Dianette®—contains an anti-androgen: cyproterone acetate.

5 If there is no improvement after 6 months, finasteride, 5 mg daily, can be tried by women who will not fall pregnant. This is well tolerated and can be used for idiopathic or polycystic ovarian hirsutism. It slows the growth of new hair.

Special points

1 A hair has a life cycle of about 2 years, so that therapy must be prolonged.

2 75% of patients will notice improvement within 6 months.

3 Postmenopausal women may develop mild hirsutism as free circulating testosterone increases. No treatment is necessary, but hormone replacement therapy (HRT) may be helpful as it increases sex hormone binding globulin and the free testosterone level falls.

4 Some investigators have suggested that 90% of women with so-called idiopathic hirsutism actually have polycystic ovaries on ultrasonic examination despite normal menstrual cycles.

Polycystic ovarian disease with hirsutism

Ovarian dysfunction characterised by increased androgen production.

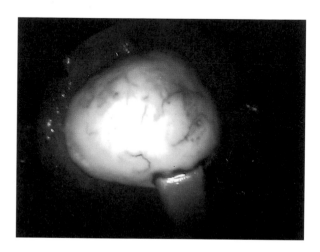

Fig 12.3 The large, pale, hyperandrogenic ovary.

Symptoms
These women have the following.
1 Irregular menstrual cycles from the menarche, but can be normal.
2 May be obese due to hyperinsulinaemia.
3 Gradual onset of hirsutism after puberty.
4 Bitemporal hairline recession and frontal thinning.
5 Infertility or miscarriage may be noted in the history.
6 Serum testosterone slightly raised: 2–5 nmol/l.
7 LH typically raised on Day 5 of cycle—over 10 IU/l, but often normal.

Polycystic ovarian disease with hirsutism

Management

Control can be achieved by the following.

1 Weight reduction if necessary to reduce hyperinsulinaemia.

2 Contraception and cycle control with Dianette®: also helps with acne.

3 Local cosmetic treatments as above.

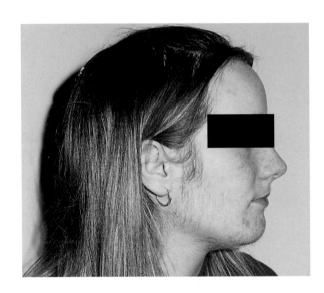

Fig 12.4 Note hair thinning and temporal baldness.

Virilisation

This is a rare condition associated with serious, life-threatening adrenal disorders and ovarian tumours, but occurs in less than 1% of women with hirsutism.

Virilisation

Symptoms

Severe degree of hyperandrogenism results in:

1 Hirsutism of recent onset and rapid development.
2 Breast reduction.
3 Cliteromegaly.
4 Deepening of the voice.
5 Secondary amenorrhoea.
6 Striae on abdomen or legs.

Investigation

Serum testosterone over 6 nmol/l.

Management

Immediate referral to specialist endocrinology clinic.

13 Recurrent miscarriage

Recurrent miscarriage, 250

Recurrent miscarriage

The most common complication of pregnancy is miscarriage. Recurrent miscarriage is defined as three or more consecutive miscarriages.

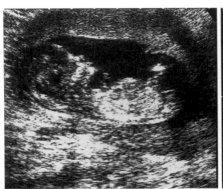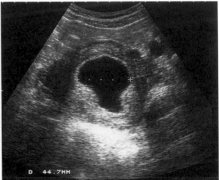

Fig 13.1 Ultrasound images of viable gestation compared with missed abortion at 10 weeks.

Incidence
1 Affects 1% of women.
2 10–20% of all clinically evident pregnancies will miscarry by 12 weeks' gestation.
3 50% of all fertilised ova are lost before pregnancy is evident.

Aetiology
Multifactorial.
1 Polycystic ovarian disease with luteinising hormone (LH) hypersecretion—20%.
2 Thrombophilic disorders—17%.
3 Uterine or cervical abnormality—12%.
4 Chromosomal abnormality—3%.
5 Hypothyroidism—1–2%.

Recurrent miscarriage

6 70% of early embryonic demise is caused by chromosomal defects which are accidental and non-repetitive.

Investigations

1 After the first miscarriage—none indicated.
   (a) Reassurance that the women has an 85% chance of a live baby in a subsequent pregnancy.
   (b) Acknowledge the grief reaction experienced by 75% of women during first month after loss.
   (c) Patient leaflet given before discharge (see p. 253).
   (d) Advise need to wait until emotionally ready before trying again.
   (e) Reassure the couple that they did not 'cause' the loss.
2 After two or more miscarriages.
   (a) Anticardiolipin antibody status: lupus anticoagulant (LA), anticardiolipin antibodies (ACA). Women with lupus may admit to migraines, epilepsy, skin rashes and arthralgia.
   (b) Karyotyping of woman and her partner for chromosomal anomaly.
   (c) Vaginal ultrasound and hysteroscopy to exclude uterine anomaly.
   (d) Infection screen, e.g. bacterial vaginosis.

Recurrent miscarriage

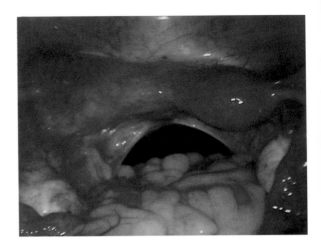

Fig 13.2 Young women with recurrent miscarriage may have uterine abnormality—double uterus seen at laparoscopy.

Management

1 The grief reaction can be severe and distressing and may take the couple many months to recover. Avoid the use of terms such as abortion and fetus.

2 'Tender loving care' and frequent visits in the subsequent first trimester have resulted in an 85% success rate in women compared with a 35% success rate in those not receiving extra care.

3 High-resolution scanning at 6 weeks' gestation can identify a fetal heart and, if beating, 98% of pregnancies will continue to term.

4 Weekly scanning during the first trimester is appropriate and reassuring.

5 Fetal growth should be monitored in these 'high-risk' women.

6 Women may be comforted by the knowledge of statistics, which show that the chance of a successful pregnancy after:

Recurrent miscarriage

(a) one miscarriage is 85%;
(b) two miscarriages is 72%;
(c) three miscarriages is 66%;
(d) four miscarriages is 59%;
(e) five miscarriages is 50%.

7 Maternal age is important as women over 30 years of age have more subfertility and an increased risk of miscarriage.

Treatment in specialist clinic

1 If antiphospholipid antibodies are present, aspirin, 75 mg daily, before and during pregnancy is advised. Heparin may be added during pregnancy.

2 Specialist units may undertake treatment of women with polycystic ovarian disease and LH hypersecretion by pituitary suppression and ovulation induction but treatment is complex and costly.

3 Genetic counselling is offered to women with karyotype abnormalities in either partner.

4 Often none as 'no cause' is identified.

Special points

1 Miscarriage clinics for support and counselling after the event are recognised to be beneficial.

2 The Miscarriage Association has patient information sheets which are helpful.

 (a) Miscarriage Association, Clayton Hospital, Northgate, Wakefield, West Yorkshire, WF1 3JS. Telephone: 01924 200 799.

 (b) SANDS (Stillbirth and Neonatal Death Society), 28 Portland Place, London, W1N 4DE. Telephone: 0171 436 7940. Helpline: 0171 436 5881 (Monday–Friday, 9.30 a.m. to 5.30 p.m.).

14 Genital cancer

Premalignant disease of the cervix

Screening to detect premalignant cervical disease is a very common gynaecological procedure.

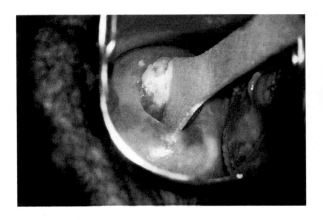

Fig 14.1 Cervical smear.

Incidence
1 21 per 100000 women develop severe dysplasia of the cervix in the UK and this is detected by cervical cytology.
2 Over a 20-year period, 40% of these lesions may progress to cervical cancer if not detected and treated.

Aetiology
Probably, human papilloma virus (HPV) infection inactivates a tumour suppressor gene (P54) and makes the woman more susceptible to oncogenic change. Risk factors include the following.
1 Multiple sexual partners.
2 Early first age of sexual intercourse.
3 Smoking.

Premalignant disease of the cervix

Screening to prevent invasive disease

1 Long prodromal period so that cytological screening of women aged 20–64 years is feasible.

2 Cervical screening rates of up to 83% had been achieved by GPs by 1993 with computerised call and recall support.

3 The NHS Cervical Screening Programme recommends routine cervical smears every 3–5 years.

Management of abnormal smear

Laboratory directs GP on patient management — repeat smear or refer for colposcopy.

Colposcopy service

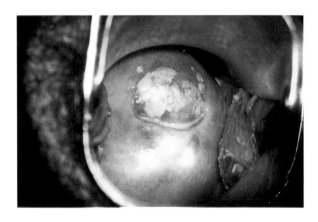

Fig 14.2 The abnormal area stained and visualised at colposcopy.

Colposcopy service

1 Procedure undertaken as an out-patient with local anaesthesia for any treatment required.

2 Cervix inspected and lesion biopsied under magnification.

3 Cervical intraepithelial neoplasia (CIN) treated by:

(a) 'cold' coagulation (heating to 100°C);

(b) large loop excision of the transformation zone (LLETZ). Occasionally, laser vaporisation or cone excision.

4 LLETZ technique provides tissue for histology and reassurance of complete excision of abnormality.

5 Secondary haemorrhage is rare, but can occur, and requires readmission to hospital and vaginal packing or treatment of bleeding point.

6 HPV infection is commonly reported on cervical smears and does not require treatment.

7 Precancerous lesions are called CIN and are graded:

(a) CIN 1—mild dysplasia;

(b) CIN 2—moderate dysplasia;

(c) CIN 3—severe dysplasia.

8 Early cervical cancer:

(a) microinvasive carcinoma—lesion penetrates the basement membrane by less than 3 mm;

(b) invasive carcinoma—lesion penetrates the basement membrane by more than 3–5 mm.

The term 'carcinoma *in situ*' is no longer used.

Colposcopy service

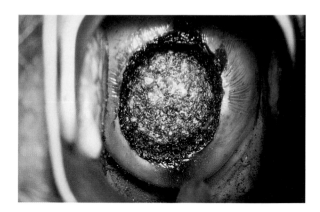

Fig 14.3 Treatment with local ablative techniques has a 90% cure rate.

9 Follow-up at discretion of clinic. Annual smears for 5 years to detect recurrence or incomplete treatment, with return to normal recall after 5 years.

10 Psychosexual problems can occur because of the nature of the condition.

Special points

Knife cone biopsy under general anaesthesia is rarely practised because of complications and scarring afterwards and the effectiveness of LLETZ.

Colposcopy service

The healed cervix after treatment

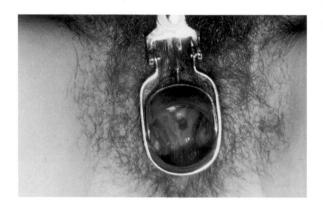

Fig 14.4 The healed cervix after treatment.

1 Destruction of the ectocervix sometimes allows the endocervix to become prominent after healing.

2 Many practitioners, seeing this, are concerned about the appearance and refer the patient again for colposcopy.

3 Protrusion or prolapse of the columnar epithelium of the endocervix is common after ablation treatment and, provided that the smear is normal, no further action is required.

Invasive cancer of the cervix

The second most common malignancy in women.

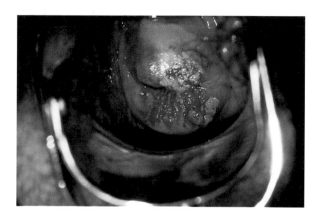

Fig 14.5 Carcinoma of the cervix.

Incidence
1 13 per 100 000 women, with bimodal incidence in the early thirties and again in the sixties.
2 The incidence and mortality have increased for women aged 25–34 years.
3 90% are squamous carcinoma.
4 10% are adenocarcinoma.

Symptoms
1 Early disease is symptomless and only detected by screening.
2 Late disease presents with:
   (a) postcoital bleeding;
   (b) postmenopausal bleeding;
   (c) offensive vaginal discharge, often bloodstained.
3 A suspicious looking cervix on routine examination.

Invasive cancer of the cervix

Diagnosis
1 Needs urgent referral for colposcopy and large biopsy to confirm.
2 Examination under anaesthesia (EUA):
    (a) to stage tumour and biopsy;
    (b) cystoscopy;
    (c) rectal examination;
    (d) IVU and chest X-ray;
    (e) computed tomography (CT) scan or magnetic resonance imaging (MRI).

Survival rate—5 years
1 Stage I localised to cervix, 80%.
2 Stage II paracervical spread, 50%.
3 Stage III pelvic spread, 25%.
4 Stage IV distant spread, 5%.

Treatment of carcinoma

Stage Ia—preclinical and microinvasive
1 Young women. Local excision with LLETZ or cone biopsy.
2 Older women. Simple hysterectomy may be more suitable.

Stage Ib or IIa—deeper cervical lesion, paracervical or into vagina
1 Wertheim's hysterectomy (radical hysterectomy) and lymphadenectomy for younger women as ovaries conserved.
2 Radiotherapy for:
    (a) older, unfit patients;
    (b) the 20% found to have lymph node involvement at surgery;
    (c) primary treatment for advanced cases.

Invasive cancer of the cervix

Advanced cases
Chemotherapy—cisplatin, methotrexate, bleomycin—may be given with response in 50% of cases before radiotherapy or surgery.

Terminal care
1 As disease escapes control or recurs, ureteral invasion occurs.
2 Local vaginal bleeding, anaemia and uraemia can develop, and either hospital- or hospice-based care with cancer nursing support is required.
3 Pain not often a problem but, in young women, death from cancer of the cervix is particularly distressing.

Useful addresses of organisations concerned with cancer care
1 Cancer BACUP, Cancer Counselling Service, 3 Bath Place, Rivington Street, London EC2A 3JR. Telephone: 0171 696 9000. Freephone: 0800 18 11 99.
2 CancerLink, 11–21 Northdown Street, London NI 9BN. Freephone: 0800 132 905.
3 Macmillan Cancer Relief, Anchor House, 15–19 Britten Street, London, SW3 3TZ. Telephone: 0171 351 7811. Information line 0845 6016 161.
4 Marie Curie Cancer Care, 28 Belgrave Square, London, SW1X 8QG. Telephone: 0171 235 3325.
5 Tak Tent Cancer Support Scotland, Block C20, Western Court, 100 University Place, Glasgow, G12 6SQ. Telephone: 0141 211 1930.
6 Tenovous Cancer Information Centre, College Buildings, Courtenay Road, Splott,

Invasive cancer of the cervix

Cardiff, CF1 1SA. Telephone: 01222 497 700. Freephone: 0800 526 527.

7 The Ulster Cancer Foundation, 40 Eglantine Avenue, Belfast, BT9 6DX. Telephone: 01232 663 281. Helpline: 01232 663 439.

8 Women's Health Information Centre, 52 Featherstone Street, London, EC1Y 8RT. Telephone: 0171 251 6580.

9 Women's Nationwide Cancer Control Campaign, Suna House, 128–130 Curtain Road, London, EC2A 3AR. Telephone: 0171 729 1735/4688.

Endometrial cancer

Abnormal bleeding is the commonest presenting symptom of endometrial cancer and 80% of women are postmenopausal.

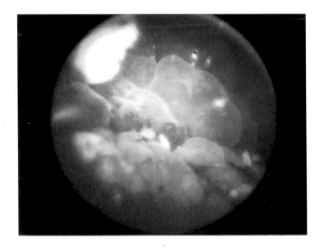

Fig 14.6 Hysteroscopic view of carcinoma in the uterus.

Endometrial cancer

Incidence
1 Rare before 45 years of age, increases up to menopause and then falls in old age.
2 Mean age of 61 years.
3 One-third of premenopausal cancers present with heavy, *regular* periods.

Aetiology
1 Related to oestrogen exposure—nulliparity, late menopause.
2 Commoner in obese women.
3 Polycystic ovarian disease—these women are hyperoestrogenised.
4 Unopposed oestrogen including ovarian tumours and tamoxifen therapy.

Symptoms
1 Menstrual irregularities.
2 Postmenopausal bleeding.
3 Abdominal fullness and pain.
4 Vaginal discharge due to pyometra.

Diagnosis
1 All postmenopausal bleeding must be investigated.
2 Vaginal spotting should not be attributed to atrophic vaginitis.
3 All patients with heavy, irregular peri-menopausal bleeds should be investigated.

Investigations
1 Pelvic ultrasound scan to check endometrial thickness (normal: less than 4 mm after the menopause).
2 Full blood count (FBC).

Endometrial cancer

3 Cervical smear.
4 Referral to specialist clinic for:
   (a) endometrial sampling;
   (b) hysteroscopy and curettage.

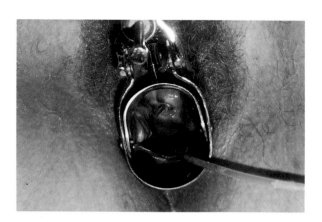

Fig 14.7 The Pipelle suction device will only miss 5% of tumours.

Management
1 Early recourse to surgery.
2 Total abdominal hysterectomy and bilateral salpingo-oophorectomy plus pelvic and para-aortic node sampling.

Special points

Most patients prefer to be told the truth about their condition.

Poor prognostic features
1 Advanced age and advanced stage.
2 Poorly differentiated tumour, especially

Endometrial cancer

clear cell tumour and serous papillary carcinoma.

3 Myometrial invasion of more than 50% of wall depth.

4 Involvement of pelvic or para-aortic nodes.

5 Tumour involving the cervix — 25% reduction in survival rate.

Survival in stage I disease

1 75% of patients present with disease confined to the uterus and only early myometrial invasion and have an excellent prognosis.

2 Stage I tumour — 5-year survival rate in excess of 80%.

Survival in late stage disease

Spread to the cervix, beyond the uterus and into the pelvis has a poor prognosis with a 5-year survival rate falling from 50% to 11% in Stage IV disease.

Postoperative radiotherapy

Indicated to whole pelvis plus treatment to vaginal vault.

Advanced or recurrent disease

1 Recurrent disease will manifest within 3 years in 70% of patients destined to have this.

2 30% of patients with endometrial cancer respond to hormonal therapy with:

    (a) medroxyprogesterone acetate — Provera®;

    (b) megestrol acetate — Megace®.

This controls the bleeding and increases the

Endometrial cancer

sense of well-being, but may not lengthen the survival time.

3 Chemotherapy may be tried in relapsed cases.

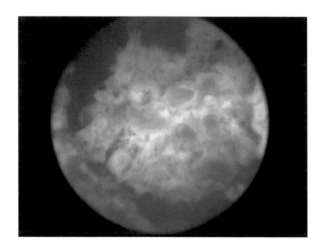

Fig 14.8 Patient used 'wild yam' for hormone replacement and presented with bleeding and tumour at hysteroscopy.

Special points

1 Endometrial cancer may run in families, and there is a link to hereditary non-polyposis colorectal cancer.

2 A family history should be taken and, if other female members have endometrial cancer, this syndrome may be present and male family members may be at risk of bowel cancer.

Ovarian cancer

The most common form of gynaecological cancer, but the average GP will only see 5–10 cases during a practising life.

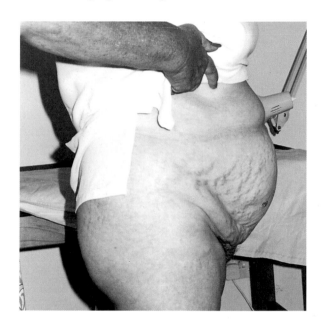

Fig 14.9 One of the most dreaded cancers known as 'The Silent Killer' and mistaken for middle-aged spread by the woman. Presents late.

Incidence
1 5000 new cases a year.
2 The fourth commonest cause of death from cancer in women and leading cause of death from gynaecological malignancy.
3 The mean age at onset is 59 years.
4 The median survival is only 2 years.
5 The 5-year survival rate is around 30%.

Aetiology
Usually unknown.
1 Mutations in P53 regulatory gene.
2 Talc particles may be implicated.

Ovarian cancer

Symptoms
1 Notoriously late, vague and non-gynaecological.
2 Abdominal distension and discomfort.
3 Bowel dysfunction and unexplained gastrointestinal symptoms.
4 Anorexia and weight loss.
5 Dyspepsia and flatulence.
6 Patient notices a mass.
7 Postmenopausal bleeding.
8 Backache, ankle oedema and thrombophlebitis.

Diagnosis
Refer *early* and *urgently* on *suspicion*.
1 Patients are usually in the advanced stage of the disease at diagnosis and have little time to prepare themselves for the consequences of the diagnosis.
2 Elderly women present with abdominal distension, cachexia and an ascitic fluid thrill.
3 Leg oedema is a late symptom.
4 Note that vaginal bleeding is not a feature.

Ovarian cancer

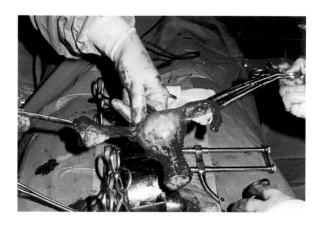

Fig 14.10 Patient aged 44 years with two children, menorrhagia and three close relatives with ovarian cancer requested total abdominal hysterectomy and bilateral salpingo-oophorectomy.

Incidence
1 Most cases are sporadic.
2 No current screening tests have proved to be reliable. Both CA125 and transvaginal ultrasound are poorly predictive for population screening.

Women with no family history of ovarian cancer
1 1% lifetime risk of the disease.
2 Pelvic examination is sufficiently specific and sensitive to be useful as a screening test.
3 Reassurance and no further action.
4 Anxious patients may demand ultrasound and a CA125 tumour marker test. Normal if under 30 U/ml.

Women with affected relatives
1 One affected first-degree relative —5% risk.
2 Two affected first-degree relatives —30% risk.
3 In 5% of all cases of ovarian cancer, there is a familial association linked with the inheritance

Ovarian cancer

of a high-risk gene, such as BRCA1 and 2. These cause site-specific ovarian cancer, cases of cancer of the breast and ovary and cases of cancer of the breast, ovary, colon or endometrium.

Close relatives of these families should be advised to undergo screening
1 Annual screening starts at 25 years of age with pelvic examination, serum CA125 and transvaginal scan.
2 Breast cancer families — mammography every 2 years from 25 years of age and yearly from 35 years of age.
3 Oral contraceptives are protective against ovarian cancer and should be advised.
4 After 35 years of age, prophylactic oophorectomy should be offered, followed by hormone replacement therapy (HRT).

Hospital management
Request *urgent* admission for investigation. This will include the following.
1 A pelvic ultrasound scan to detect pelvic masses, ascites.
2 Assessment of the renal tract by scan or intravenous pyelography.
3 Blood count and serum albumen.
4 Tumour marker assays, e.g. CA125, inhibin.
5 Paracentesis for cytology.

Treatment
1 Radical abdominal surgery will include:
   (a) total abdominal hysterectomy, bilateral

Ovarian cancer

salpingo-oophorectomy, omentectomy and tumour debulking;

(b) bowel resection may be indicated.

2 Chemotherapy:

(a) adjuvant therapy with six cycles at monthly intervals of carboplatin or cisplatin;

(b) taxanes and topotecan in relapsing cases.

Prognosis

1 Stage I disease — 95% 5-year survival rate.

2 Stage IV disease — 10% 5-year survival rate.

Multidisciplinary management

1 GP, surgeon, oncologist, cancer nurses and hospice.

2 Counselling of relatives best done by GP, and good liaison between GP and hospital is central to the management.

3 The cancer nurse is often the 'lifeline' to the woman and provides compassion and continuity of care.

4 Chemotherapy courses can give rise to symptoms of nausea, gastrointestinal problems and depression, and the patient will turn to the GP for support.

5 Patients may be entered into drug trials, e.g. ICON, $ICON_3$, $ICON_4$.

Centres for screening and advice

Patients may be referred to the following centres for screening and advice.

1 CRC, Department of Oncology, Cambridge Institute for Medical Research, Box 139, Addenbrookes Hospital, Hills Road,

Ovarian cancer

Cambridge CB2 2XY. Telephone: 01223 336 900.

2 Randomised Trial of Screening for Ovarian Cancer, Ovarian Cancer Screening Unit, Royal Hospitals Trust, St Bartholomew's Hospital, London, EC1A 7BE. Telephone: 0171 706 7651. Fax: 0171 601 7652.

15 Hysterectomy and transcervical resection of the endometrium (TCRE)

Hysterectomy

The commonest major operation performed on women.

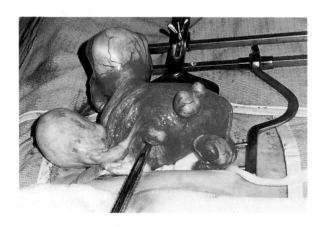

Fig 15.1 Heavy, painful periods cause many women to seek a hysterectomy.

Incidence
70 000 women undergo hysterectomy each year in the UK.

Aetiology
1 Menorrhagia, 50%.
2 Prolapse, 20%.
3 Pain from pelvis or pelvic pathology, 20%.
4 Cancer, 10%.

Counselling
1 Most women have tried various alternative treatments for their condition under guidance from their GP and hospital specialist for some time before considering a hysterectomy as a solution to the problem.
2 When surgery is advised in the specialist clinic, the woman may go back to consult her

Hysterectomy

GP to discuss the matter fully to understand the postoperative course.

3 The oral contraceptive pill should be stopped 4 weeks before surgery and other methods of contraception used.

4 Hormone replacement therapy (HRT) may be continued provided that there is no previous history of thromboembolism and a short surgical stay is anticipated.

5 Weight loss is essential for overweight women, as obesity increases surgical difficulty and postoperative morbidity.

6 The woman may be offered oophorectomy at the time of her hysterectomy, and the reasons for this, as well as the advantages and disadvantages of ovarian removal, must be discussed and consent obtained. Many women have strong views on retaining their own hormonal balance.

7 There is no convincing evidence, as yet, that hysterectomy reduces orgasmic intensity or frequency, and sexual activity after the operation can be as at the preoperative level.

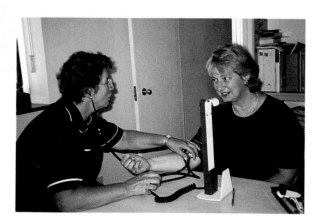

Fig 15.2 Examining woman in clinic.

Hysterectomy

Pre-admission clinics

1 These are increasingly common to check women in before surgery and to undertake special investigations, e.g. electrocardiogram (ECG), chest X-ray in the sick and elderly. Blood is cross-matched.

2 Consent forms are very important and co-signatories should be surgeons involved in the procedures who can give adequate information to obtain informed consent and advise on risks and complications.

3 It is recommended that the surgeon undertaking the procedure obtains the woman's consent.

4 Advice on ward protocols and suggested admission times are explained.

The day of surgery

1 The anaesthetist will visit the woman to check on medical fitness, drugs and allergies and will discuss the type of anaesthetic, e.g. epidural or spinal with inhalational anaesthetic. Women can be assured that they will be asleep.

2 Food and drink is withheld and limited pubic shaving is undertaken.

3 Prophylactic antibiotics are routinely administered in most units, often with the pre-medication drugs.

4 Women over 40 years of age and others with risk factors for thromboembolism are given prophylactic anticoagulation, usually subcutaneons heparin.

5 Urinary catheterisation for 24 h after surgery can increase postoperative comfort, as

Hysterectomy

sedation may cause loss of sensation of bladder filling and restlessness.

6 A patient-controlled analgesia (PCA) unit is often used and allows the self-administration of morphine sulphate in short, frequent 'press button' bursts. Safety mechanisms to prevent overdosage are incorporated.

7 Postoperative nausea is common, and drugs such as metoclopramide (Maxolon®) or ondansetron (Zofran®) can be used.

8 Early mobilisation is encouraged.

9 Oral fluids are commenced when bowel sounds can be heard and the intravenous (IV) drip has been removed.

10 Eating and bowel activity should be normal before discharge.

11 Most women have sutures removed about Day 5 and are discharged home in 5–7 days.

Post-hysterectomy advice

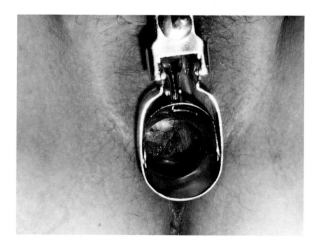

Fig 15.3 Vault granulations post-hysterectomy.

Hysterectomy

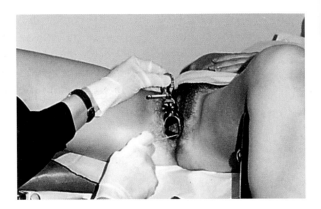

Fig 15.4 Cauterisation of vault granulations.

1 The first month at home is used for convalescence and adequate rest is recommended.
2 Driving can resume after about 1 month.
3 Slight weight gain owing to reduced activity may occur, but hysterectomy as such does *not* lead to weight gain. Within 3–6 months, weight should be back to normal as activity reverts to normal.
4 Fatigue and loss of stamina are common, but should be short term.
5 A postoperative check is performed 6 weeks after surgery by the gynaecologist.
6 Sexual intercourse can resume after this check and should feel normal with the usual orgasmic frequency.
7 Vault granulations may cause some postcoital bleeding and can be cauterised with a silver nitrate stick in the clinic or surgery.
8 Occasionally, a vault infection may occur and

Hysterectomy

manifests by an unpleasant vaginal discharge. It can be treated with an antibiotic that covers anaerobes, e.g. metronidazole.

9 A recuperative period of 6 weeks is usually recommended, after which the woman can return to work.

Results of hysterectomy

Morbidity of hysterectomy

Minor postoperative complications occur in 40% of abdominal hysterectomies and 25% of vaginal hysterectomies.

1 Postoperative pyrexia, 30%.
2 Urinary tract infections, 8%.
3 Wound infection, 4%.
4 Pulmonary embolism, 0.7%.
5 Secondary haemorrhage, 0.6%.

Mortality of hysterectomy

1 Abdominal hysterectomy, 86 per 100 000.
2 Vaginal hysterectomy, 27 per 100 000.

Special points

1 96% of women are satisfied with the results of their operation and felt the decision to undergo surgery was correct.
2 50% of women with preoperative psychiatric morbidity showed mood improvement and better psychosexual and social functioning after the procedure.

Hysterectomy

Postoperative ovarian failure

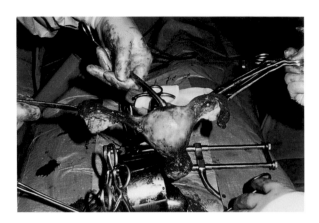

Fig 15.5 Removal of ovaries necessitates HRT counselling.

1 Women who have had their ovaries removed should be offered oestrogen replacement therapy at the time of surgery and the implications discussed.

2 Ovarian failure can occur earlier in women who undergo a hysterectomy with ovarian conservation.

3 Women should be educated to recognise the symptoms of hot flushes and vaginal dryness so that treatment options can be discussed.

Types of hysterectomy

**Vaginal
hysterectomy**

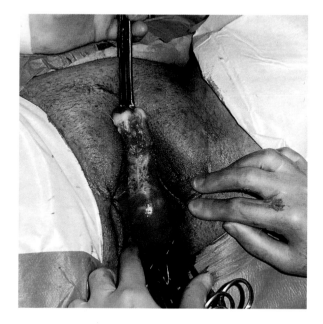

Fig 15.6 The 'natural' exit route for the organ.

Characteristics

1 The 'gold standard' hysterectomy.

2 Ideal for parous women.

3 No abdominal wound and minimal disturbance of bowel function.

4 Excellent postoperative recovery with early mobility as no scar pain.

5 Minimal blood loss.

6 Ovaries can be removed in most cases.

7 Lower postoperative morbidity and mortality.

8 Only 30% performed in this way and should be more.

Types of hysterectomy

Total abdominal hysterectomy

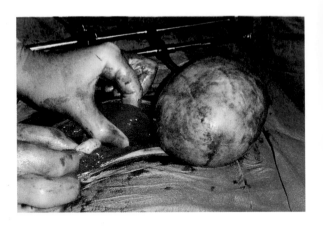

Fig 15.7 Total abdominal hysterectomy—ovarian pathology.

Characteristics

1 Used when uterus enlarged, ovarian pathology is present, in extensive endometriosis and in cancer cases where good exposure is essential for staging and radical surgery.

2 Healing of abdominal incision delays mobility and is more painful.

3 Higher incidence of postoperative morbidity and mortality, especially in obese women.

4 Still the preferred route of many gynaecologists.

Subtotal hysterectomy

Characteristics

1 Was very popular in the past.

2 The fundus of the uterus is removed leaving the cervix and the uterine arteries supplying it behind.

3 The fear of stump cancer is now obsolete with good cytological screening.

4 May preserve sexual function, but role of cervix in orgasm is not clear.

Types of hysterectomy

5 Can be done laparoscopically, but technique still under review.

Laparoscopically assisted vaginal hysterectomy

Characteristics

1 Used in women without much uterine descent.

2 Laparoscopically, the upper ligaments around the ovary and lateral uterine supports are cut with diathermy or staples to allow the uterus to descend.

3 The operation is completed with a vaginal hysterectomy along conventional lines.

4 Longer operative procedure and can be more expensive.

5 Earlier discharge from hospital may be possible.

6 Good results in experienced hands with low complication rate.

7 Less pain and postoperative analgesia.

8 Only 4–8% of hysterectomies are performed by this method in the UK.

Transcervical resection of the endometrium (TCRE)

A newer technique for the treatment of menorrhagia becoming more popular and commonly offered as an alternative to hysterectomy.

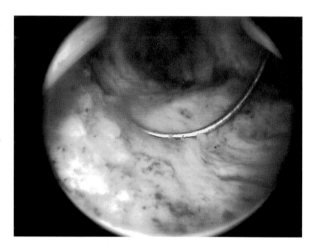

Fig 15.8 15 000 endometrial resections are performed in the UK each year.

Indications

1 Menorrhagic women who have failed to respond to medical treatment and have no significant pathology, i.e. dysfunctional uterine bleeding.

2 An alternative to hysterectomy where this operation is inconvenient because of the requirement of prolonged convalescence or dangerous because of obesity or adhesions.

3 Patient preference to retain her uterus.

4 Patient preference for quicker recovery period than hysterectomy.

Transcervical resection of the endometrium (TCRE)

Patient selection

1 Women over 35 years of age with significant menorrhagia.

2 Family completed as fertility will be affected.

3 Pathology, e.g. cancer, must be excluded.

4 Significant fibroids should not be present. Small ones can be safely resected.

Technique

1 Under a general anaesthetic, the endometrium is removed by electrical diathermy, roller ball or laser ablation.

2 Small islands of endometrium can remain and subsequently proliferate.

3 Haemorrhage, perforation and fluid overload are rare complications and relate to operator experience.

4 HRT, if required, should be with a continuous combined preparation, e.g. Climesse®, Premique®, Kliofem®.

5 Pregnancies have been reported, so clip sterilisation can be offered at the time of surgery.

6 Endometrial thinning with the oral contraceptive pill or danazol prior to resection depends on the operator's and woman's preference. Results are the same whether or not this has been undertaken.

7 Postmenstrual resection is easier surgically than premenstrual resection.

Transcervical resection of the endometrium (TCRE)

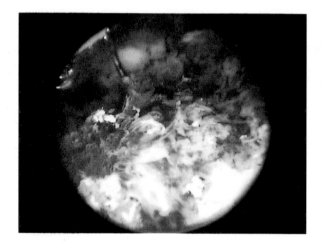

Fig 15.9 The fluffy, red endometrium is 'reamed' away with the electrical loop.

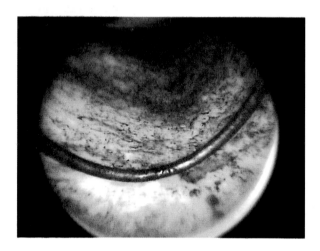

Fig 15.10 The pared and desiccated myometrium.

Results

Endometrial resection is an acceptable alternative to hysterectomy for the treatment of menorrhagia in selected cases.

Transcervical resection of the endometrium (TCRE)

1 Satisfaction rates of 80% reported in Royal College of Obstetricians and Gynaecologists 'Mistlctoe' Audit.

2 More than 50% of women continue to have reduced menstrual flow for up to 5 years after surgery.

3 Pelvic pain can occur. It is sharp and stabbing and may be caused by haematosalpinx.

4 20% of women will eventually need further surgery, usually a hysterectomy, because of:

    (a) continuing menorrhagia, usually from adenomyosis, deeply infiltrating the endometrium;

    (b) pain from haematometra or cornual bleeding;

    (c) return of menses again after some time.

5 Destruction of endometrium around the thin cornual areas of the uterus can be difficult and the roller ball can be used.

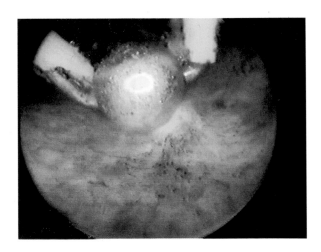

Fig 15.11 The roller ball achieves good results.

Transcervical resection of the endometrium (TCRE)

6 Amenorrhoea can occur in about 30% of patients and more if women are peri-menopausal. Oligomenorrhoea or acceptable 'normal' periods occur in the other 60% of patients.

7 Further suppression of residual endometrium may be achieved by fitting a levonorgestrel intrauterine system (IUS) (Mirena®) after surgery.

Special points

---

1 Patients should be advised to expect a bloodstained discharge for 3–4 weeks after a resection and antibiotic cover may be given for a week.

2 Postmenopausal bleeding in women who have undergone TCRE must be investigated by hysteroscopy and biopsy.

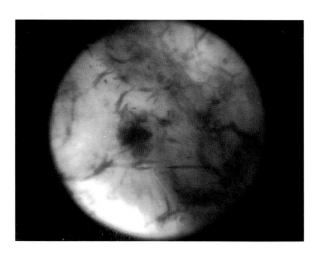

Fig 15.12 Hysteroscopic view of postresection endometrium in woman with postmenopausal bleeding.

Transcervical resection of the endometrium (TCRE)

3 Endometrial atrophy with obliteration of the cavity and adhesions are common, but carcinoma can develop in residual islands of endometrium.

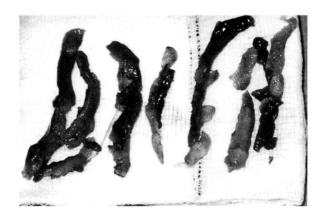

Fig 15.13 The long, resected strips contain pink endometrium and 4–5 mm of pale myometrium.

16   Breast disorders

Breast pain

So common that 70% of women attending for breast screening report cyclical breast pain.

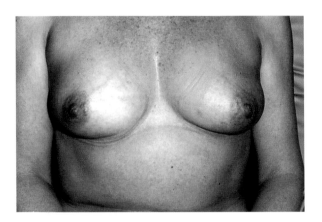

Fig 16.1 Heavy premenstrual breasts with blue veins.

Incidence
The GP may see around 30 new cases a year.

Aetiology
1 Hormonally induced and worse premenstrually.
2 Musculoskeletal chest wall pain can arise.

Cyclical breast pain

Incidence
Accounts for 45% of cases of breast pain.

Symptoms
1 Bilateral pain.
2 Upper outer quadrants.
3 Tender to the touch.
4 Heavy breasts with blue veins.
5 Worse premenstrually — third to fourth decade.

Breast pain

Management

1 Examine to exclude a discrete mass.

2 Explanation and reassurance that it is not breast cancer.

3 Breast pain chart for 3 months to check cyclical occurrence.

4 Only 15% of women will then require drug treatment.

5 Drug treatment if severe symptoms:
 (a) gamolenic acid (Efamast®), 320 mg daily in eight doses;
 (b) bromocriptine, 1.25 mg daily building up to 2.5 mg twice daily for 6 months;
 (c) danazol, 100 mg twice daily and, when responds, reduce to 100 mg daily for 7 days premenstrually;
 (d) tamoxifen, 10 mg daily in refractory cases;
 (e) goserelin implants, 3.5 mg subcutaneously monthly for severe recurrent or refractory cases only.

6 Pyridoxine, diuretics and progestogens are of no proven value.

7 Review therapy in 2 months with symptom chart.

8 Continue treatment for 6 months. If response is poor, change the drug. Danazol has a high response rate as a second-line drug.

Special points

1 If pain recurs after treatment, patient may not request further treatment.

2 Reassurance about breast cancer and a mammogram are sufficient for most patients.

Non-cyclical breast pain

Incidence

Accounts for 25% of cases of breast pain.

Breast pain

Management

1 Severe cases need referral to a specialist clinic for diagnosis, e.g. Tietze's syndrome and to reassure the patient. Less severe or intermittent cases can be offered:

    (a) non-steroidal anti-inflammatory drugs (NSAIDs);

    (b) gamolenic acid (Efamast®) can be used as first-line therapy as few side effects, but can be expensive;

    (c) danazol is the most effective drug, but the side effects may limit use.

2 Refer to specialist breast surgeon if patient has:

    (a) unilateral persistent pain in post-menopausal women;

    (b) intractable pain not responding to above management;

    (c) pain associated with a lump.

3 Further investigation in specialist clinic:

    (a) mammography;

    (b) ultrasonography;

    (c) fine needle aspiration cytology if appropriate.

Breast lumps

Breast cancer is the commonest malignant condition to affect women.

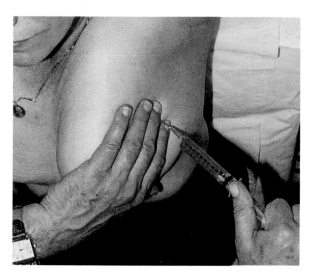

Fig 16.2 Fine needle aspiration of breast cyst in outpatient clinic.

Incidence

1 A common cause for consultation with the GP in all age groups.

2 Breast cancer is the commonest condition to affect women, with a 1 : 12 lifetime risk of developing the disease.

3 Found at self-examination, during washing and on mammography screening in women over 50 years of age.

4 Mammographic screening is used to identify women with ductal carcinoma *in situ* which is considered to be a premalignant condition and wide local excision is indicated.

5 20% of breast cancer patients are premenopausal and mammography is not as successful in this younger group in reducing mortality.

Breast lumps

6 Common histological groups:
 (a) fibroadenosis, 75%;
 (b) cystic change, 15%;
 (c) carcinoma, 6%;
 (d) fibroadenoma, 3%.

Management
1 Examine the patient.
2 If there is no lump palpable, reassure but request return visit to reassess in a month.
3 Surveillance can be undertaken by the GP in:
 (a) young women with tender, lumpy breasts which fluctuate with the menstrual cycle;
 (b) older women with diffusely nodular breasts provided that no discrete lesion develops;
 (c) recurrent multiple cysts previously diagnosed as benign can be aspirated by the GP with the necessary skills.
4 Referral to a specialist breast service is recommended if:
 (a) a discrete breast lump is present;
 (b) a new discrete lump develops in preexisting nodularity;
 (c) asymmetrical nodularity persists at review after menstruation;
 (d) an abscess is present;
 (e) there is persistent refilling or recurrent cyst;
 (f) there is a change in the skin contour;
 (g) a woman with a strong family history of breast cancer requests assessment.
Any woman over 35 years of age with a discrete breast lump should be referred for mammography.

Breast lumps

5 Management in the specialist clinic is by triple assessment:
  (a) clinical examination;
  (b) imaging—ultrasound or mammography;
  (c) fine needle aspiration cytology or core biopsy with Trucut.

Special points about breast cancer

1 In the UK, there are 26 000 new cases of breast cancer each year.

2 Breast cancer is the biggest cancer killer amongst women, with approximately 16 000 deaths each year in the UK.

3 The UK has the highest mortality rate in the world.

4 British women have the worst prognosis in Europe, with a 5-year survival rate of only 60% compared with the European rate of 66%. The 5-year survival rate for Stage 1 disease is 84% and for Stage 4 disease is 18%.

5 The National Breast Screening Programme aims to provide mammography for all women aged 50 years and over. Mammography has been shown to have the highest sensitivity and specificity of any of the breast imaging tests currently available. Two-yearly screening should be introduced and two screens in later years to age 69 years have been recommended.

6 Women genetically predisposed to breast cancer often request mammographic screening.

7 Women should be warned that there is no proven benefit, and that the cumulative radiation dose might result in the risk outweighing the benefit.

Nipple discharge

Common in women on oral contraceptives or with hyperprolactinaemia and women who squeeze their nipples to 'check' for discharge.

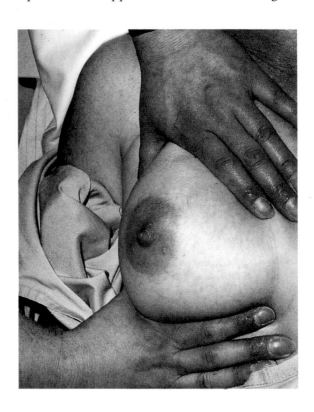

Fig 16.3 Clear nipple discharge is usually innocuous but can indicate underlying pathology.

Management
1 Take a history of the extent of discharge and the presence of blood staining.
2 Examine the breast for a lump and whether a single duct or multiple ducts are discharging.
3 Refer to a specialist breast clinic if:
    (a) the woman is 50 years of age or over;
    (b) a breast lump is also present;

Nipple discharge

Special points

Breast examination is an integral part of the gynae-cological examination and the gynaecologist may be the first clini-cian to detect a breast disorder.

(c) there is bilateral discharge staining clothes;

(d) blood staining is present;

(e) there is persistent single duct discharge;

(f) the nipple is distorted, retracted or eczematous.

4 Mammography and/or ultrasound will be arranged in the specialist clinic.

5 The GP can keep under surveillance the pre-menopausal woman with a clear discharge that is from multiple ducts and is intermittent.

Index

Page references in *italics* refer to figures; those in **bold** refer to tables